21st CENTURY MEDICINE: HOW TELEHEALTH CAN HELP RURAL COMMUNITIES

HEARING

BEFORE THE

SUBCOMMITTEES ON AGRICULTURE, ENERGY, AND TRADE AND HEALTH AND TECHNOLOGY

OF THE

COMMITTEE ON SMALL BUSINESS UNITED STATES HOUSE OF REPRESENTATIVES

ONE HUNDRED FIFTEENTH CONGRESS

FIRST SESSION

HEARING HELD
JULY 20, 2017

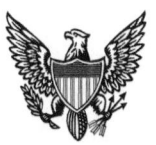

Small Business Committee Document Number 115–031
Available via the GPO Website: www.fdsys.gov

U.S. GOVERNMENT PUBLISHING OFFICE
26–251   WASHINGTON : 2017

For sale by the Superintendent of Documents, U.S. Government Publishing Office
Internet: bookstore.gpo.gov   Phone: toll free (866) 512–1800; DC area (202) 512–1800
Fax: (202) 512–2104   Mail: Stop IDCC, Washington, DC 20402–0001

HOUSE COMMITTEE ON SMALL BUSINESS

STEVE CHABOT, Ohio, *Chairman*
STEVE KING, Iowa
BLAINE LUETKEMEYER, Missouri
DAVE BRAT, Virginia
AUMUA AMATA COLEMAN RADEWAGEN, American Samoa
STEVE KNIGHT, California
TRENT KELLY, Mississippi
ROD BLUM, Iowa
JAMES COMER, Kentucky
JENNIFFER GONZALEZ-COLON, Puerto Rico
DON BACON, Nebraska
BRIAN FITZPATRICK, Pennsylvania
ROGER MARSHALL, Kansas
RALPH NORMAN, South Carolina
NYDIA VELÁZQUEZ, New York, *Ranking Member*
DWIGHT EVANS, Pennsylvania
STEPHANIE MURPHY, Florida
AL LAWSON, JR., Florida
YVETTE CLARK, New York
JUDY CHU, California
ALMA ADAMS, North Carolina
ADRIANO ESPAILLAT, New York
BRAD SCHNEIDER, Illinois
VACANT

KEVIN FITZPATRICK, *Majority Staff Director*
JAN OLIVER, *Majority Deputy Staff Director and Chief Counsel*
ADAM MINEHARDT, *Staff Director*

CONTENTS

OPENING STATEMENTS

	Page
Hon. Rod Blum	1
Hon. Brad Schneider	2
Hon. Al Lawson	3
Hon. Trent Kelly	4

WITNESSES

Ms. A. Nicole Clowers, Managing Director, Health Care Team, United States Government Accountability Office, Washington, DC 5
Ms. Barb Johnston, Chief Executive Officer and Co-Founder, HealthLinkNow, Sacramento, CA 6
Mr. Michael Adcock, Administrator, Center for Telehealth, University of Mississippi Medical Center, Jackson, MS 8
David Schmitz, M.D., President, National Rural Health Association, Washington, DC 10

APPENDIX

Prepared Statements:
  Ms. A. Nicole Clowers, Managing Director, Health Care Team, United States Government Accountability Office, Washington, DC 32
  Ms. Barb Johnston, Chief Executive Officer and Co-Founder, HealthLinkNow, Sacramento, CA 43
  Mr. Michael Adcock, Administrator, Center for Telehealth, University of Mississippi Medical Center, Jackson, MS 49
  David Schmitz, M.D., President, National Rural Health Association, Washington, DC 53
Questions for the Record:
  None.
Answers for the Record:
  None.
Additional Material for the Record:
  CCA - Competitive Carriers Association 62
  GAO Report 65
  The National Congress of American Indians and The National Indian Health Board 137

21st CENTURY MEDICINE: HOW TELEHEALTH CAN HELP RURAL COMMUNITIES

THURSDAY, JULY 20, 2017

House of Representatives,
Committee on Small Business,
Subcommittee on Agriculture, Energy and Trade,
Joint with the
Subcommittee on Health and Technology,
Washington, DC.

The Subcommittees met, pursuant to call, at 10:00 a.m., in Room 2360, Rayburn House Office Building, Hon. Rod Blum [chairman of the Subcommittee] presiding.

Present: Representatives Chabot, Luetkemeyer, Radewagen, Kelly, Blum, Comer, González-Colón, Bacon, Fitzpatrick, Marshall, Lawson, Espaillat, and Schneider.

Chairman BLUM. Good morning. I call this hearing to order. The Subcommittees are here today to examine how the expansion of telehealth services may benefit small businesses and rural communities. Telehealth or telemedicine refers to the use of online video or telephone communication to deliver healthcare services that are to replace or supplement existing healthcare services.

Telehealth is becoming a vital component of medical treatment, particularly in areas where there are provider shortages, such as rural areas where I am from, or for conditions that require regular monitoring.

While 20 percent of Americans live in rural areas, only 9 percent of physicians practice there. Rural communities often struggle with provider shortages, requiring patients and their families to travel long distances to access medical care.

Telehealth may allow rural physicians to expand their patient base and to keep dollars in the community, benefitting other local small businesses, such as retail establishments and restaurants, contributing to a sense of community that American small towns pride themselves on. Expanding use of telehealth services may even attract physicians to open or relocate practices in rural areas without worrying about having enough local patients to stay in business. Those of us from rural areas would not want to live anywhere else, yet new physicians often have concerns about opening a viable practice in a rural community.

Our witnesses today will discuss the current use of telehealth and the barriers that are providing wider use. I want to thank all of them for being here today. We look forward to hearing your testimony. And I now yield to the ranking member of the Subcommittee on Agriculture, Energy, and Trade, Mr. Schneider, right on cue, for his opening statement.

Mr. SCHNEIDER. Thank you, and I am sorry I am late. Elevators. Anyway, I want to thank the panelists for being here and taking the time to share your thoughts with us about healthcare coverage for rural America.

Today, rural populations are more likely to be poorer, sicker, older, and have higher rates of uninsured compared with urban populations. Exacerbating these issues, rural Americans experience many difficulties in accessing healthcare services which leads to higher morbidity and mortality rates compared to those of their urban counterparts.

Among the primary challenges rural communities face is a lack of adequate insurance coverage or even getting coverage at all. Nearly one-quarter of all adults in rural communities are uninsured, and nearly 60 percent of the rural uninsured are low-income families.

Rural populations are less likely to have employer-sponsored health insurance. Consequently, Medicaid is a critical lifeline for rural and underserved communities. This is why efforts to repeal the progress the Affordable Care Act has made to provide coverage to underserved and rural communities is so misguided.

In addition, there is a shortage of doctors and hospitals in rural areas, and institutional barriers can make providing care in these areas especially challenging. These challenges not only result in poor health outcomes for people in rural communities but have significant implications for the local economy.

I look forward to hearing testimony today about policies that can increase the number of physicians in underserved communities and leverage technological innovation to improve health access and quality. Policies that increase insurance coverage not only benefit patients but also create jobs in the healthcare sector, a sector that is overwhelmingly comprised of small businesses.

In fact, it is estimated that, since 2012, 50,000 jobs were added to the healthcare sector as a direct result of the expansion of coverage under the Affordable Care Act. Despite this growth, there still remains a significant provider shortage in rural areas. Even with insurance coverage, many patients in rural areas struggle to find care, especially when it comes time to visit a specialist.

The fact is made abundantly clear by the ongoing opioid epidemic currently plaguing our Nation. It's estimated that as many as 3 million people in the U.S. are suffering from opioid addiction related to prescription drugs and heroin. As opioid-related deaths have gone up across the Nation, the largest increases are reported in heavily rural States. Our constituents and their families need help, but they often have no place to go. For example, 13 percent of rural communities have no behavioral health providers. Telehealth has the potential to bring high quality behavioral health services to these suffering communities.

Indeed, studies have shown that video telehealth users have satisfaction levels and outcomes similar to those clients receiving in-person therapy. Although it is still in its early stages, telehealth is expanding at a rapid rate, and has potential to dramatically improve access to quality care in a number of areas. Telehealth also has the potential to draw more doctors into practice in rural settings, who would otherwise feel isolated, and can be used to connect specialists with community providers, allowing practitioners to join a virtual community where they can receive mentoring and grow professionally.

Improving access to care in rural areas also benefits the local small business economy. There are over 1,500 rural hospitals nationwide that support nearly 2 million jobs. Every dollar spent by a rural hospital produces $2.29 of economic activities. When patients can receive care in their community, they do not need to travel to urban centers. They are able to keep their dollars within their own community and help to drive the success of local small firms. I look forward to hearing testimony today about how we can advance policies and leverage telehealth to improve access to quality healthcare for rural and underserved communities.

With that, I say thank you, and I yield back.

Chairman BLUM. Thank you, Mr. Schneider.

I would now like to yield to the ranking member of the Subcommittee on Health and Technology, Mr. Lawson, for his opening statement.

Mr. LAWSON. Thank you, Mr. Chairman, and welcome to the Committee.

Nineteen percent of the U.S. population live in rural areas, as most of you know, yet only about 9 or 10 percent of physicians practice in rural areas. Rural populations have fewer hospitals and healthcare providers, particularly specialists, than any other urban counterparts. And patients often must travel long distances, as we heard earlier, to access care while primary care providers struggle to coordinate care with specialists.

This not only has implications for doctors, clinics, and small hospitals, but for the local small business economy. However, innovations in technology are helping to alleviate the strain on small providers. Today's hearing will offer an opportunity to examine ways that we can improve access to healthcare in rural areas.

Telehealth has the potential to advance healthcare quality by reducing costs. It can save patients time and money in traveling to see their doctors while also allowing small practices to broaden their scope. This also indirectly benefits local small business economy by keeping dollars in the community to make rural areas more attractive.

I myself grew up in a rural area. And in recent years, innovations have made telehealth technology more accessible to rural providers than ever before. However, obstacles to its adoption remain. Some barriers are easy to overcome, such as educating doctors and patients about its utility. Other obstacles, such as a lack of broadband connectivity, are more challenging.

I am pleased this hearing will provide the opportunity for us to examine not only the barriers to health faced by rural communities but how innovations in technology can improve them. I hope that this hearing will help us identify ways we can encourage greater adoption of telehealth and how improved access to care benefits small business economy. I want to thank our witnesses again who traveled here today for both their participation and insight into this important topic.

With that, Mr. Chairman, I yield back.

Chairman BLUM. Thank you, Mr. Lawson.

If Committee members have an opening statement prepared, I ask that it be submitted for the record.

I would like to take a moment to explain the timing lights to our panelists. You will each have 5 minutes to deliver your testimony. The light will start out as green. When you have 1 minute remaining, the light will turn yellow. And, finally, at the end of your 5 minutes, it will turn red, and we ask that you try to adhere to that time limit to the extent possible.

I would now like to formally introduce our witnesses today. Our first witness is Ms. Nikki Clowers, the managing director of the healthcare team at the U.S. Government Accountability Office, or better known as GAO. The healthcare team at GAO recently released a report entitled "Telehealth and Remote Patient Monitoring Use in Medicare and Selected Federal Programs" and surveyed a wide variety of stakeholders on the state of telehealth use in Federal health programs. Thank you for being here with us today.

Our next witness is Ms. Barb Johnston, the chief executive officer and cofounder of HealthLinkNow in Sacramento, California. Ms. Johnston's company helps mental health providers incorporate telehealth services into their practices. Additionally, through a Centers for Medicare and Medicaid Services grant, her company integrated telehealth services into more than 80 primary care clinics in three rural States, Montana, Wyoming, and Washington. We appreciate your testimony and being here today.

And I now yield to Mr. Kelly, a member of the full Committee, for the introduction of our next witness.

Mr. KELLY. Thank you, Mr. Chairman.

I would also like to just acknowledge that the chairman of the full Committee, Chairman Chabot, has joined us, and we thank him for being here on this important event.

Thank you. I am proud to introduce Mr. Michael Adcock, the administrator of the Center for Telehealth at the University of Mississippi Medical Center, or UMMC. As executive director for UMMC Center for Telehealth, Michael is on the front lines of combating the severe doctor shortage that Mississippi faces. The UMCC Center for Telehealth is, in my opinion, the best in the country and leverages location within Mississippi's only teaching hospital to deliver high-quality care to rural patients that often lack access.

Mr. Adcock, I am excited to have a great Mississippian here today, and I look forward to hearing your opening statement.

Thank you, Mr. Chairman. I yield back.

Chairman BLUM. Thank you, Mr. Kelly.

I now yield to our ranking member, Mr. Schneider, for the introduction of our next witness.

Mr. SCHNEIDER. I am going the yield to my colleague Mr. Lawson.

Mr. LAWSON. Thank you, sir. Okay. I have the pleasure of introducing Dr. Schmitz, president of the National Rural Health Association, professor and chair in the Department of Family and Community Medicine at University of North Dakota School of Medicine and Health Sciences.

Dr. Schmitz has spent nearly 20 years in rural practice and teaching residents and students in the area of medical education, rural health, and workforce research. He is an active in both the American Academy of Family Physicians, serving on the Commission on Quality and Practice, the Global Association of Family Physicians serving as the North American representative to the executive of the Group of Rural Practices. I welcome Dr. Schmitz.

Chairman BLUM. Thank you, Mr. Lawson.

I would like to now recognize Ms. Clowers for her 5-minute testimony.

STATEMENTS OF A. NICOLE CLOWERS, MANAGING DIRECTOR, HEALTH CARE TEAM, UNITED STATES GOVERNMENT ACCOUNTABILITY OFFICE, WASHINGTON, D.C.; BARB JOHNSTON, CHIEF EXECUTIVE OFFICER AND COFOUNDER, HEALTHLINKNOW, SACRAMENTO, CALIFORNIA; MICHAEL ADCOCK, ADMINISTRATOR, CENTER FOR TELEHEALTH, UNIVERSITY OF MISSISSIPPI MEDICAL CENTER, JACKSON, MISSISSIPPI; AND DAVID SCHMITZ, M.D., PRESIDENT, NATIONAL RURAL HEALTH ASSOCIATION, WASHINGTON, D.C.

STATEMENT OF A. NICOLE CLOWERS

Ms. CLOWERS. Chairman Blum, Ranking Members Schneider and Lawson, Chairman Chabot, and members of the Subcommittee, thank you for inviting me here today to discuss our April 2017 report on telehealth.

Access to healthcare services can be challenging for some people, such as those who live in remote areas. Telehealth can provide an alternative to healthcare provided in person or at a doctor's office—for example, by providing clinical care remotely through two-way video.

In my comments today, I will cover three topics from our April report. One, the extent to which telehealth is used in Medicare and Medicaid; two, factors that affect the use of telehealth in Medicare; and, three, the different payment and delivery models that could affect the potential use of telehealth in Medicare.

First, we found that Medicare providers used telehealth services for a small proportion of beneficiaries and relatively few services. For example, an analysis of Medicare claims data by the Medicare Payment Advisory Commission, or MedPAC, shows that less than 1 percent of all Medicare Part B fee-for-service beneficiaries accessed services using telehealth in 2014.

According to MedPAC, beneficiaries using telehealth averaged about three telehealth visits in 2014, and Medicare spent about $14 million in total in telehealth services in that year. The most common telehealth visits were for evaluation and management services, followed by behavioral health services. MedPAC's analysis shows that 10 States accounted for almost half of all Medicare telehealth visits.

For Medicaid, the use of telehealth varies by State, as individual States have the option to determine whether to cover telehealth and what types of telehealth services to cover, among other things. We reviewed six States to gauge the extent to which telehealth is used by Medicaid. We found that officials from States that were generally more rural than urban said they used telehealth more frequently than officials from more urban States.

For example, Montana officials told us that they have used telehealth as a tool to help patients see both in-state and out-of-state specialists remotely, as there is a limited access to specialists in the State.

In contrast, officials from Illinois, which contains more urban areas, told us that telehealth represented a very small portion of their Medicaid budget and was used primarily to provide behavioral health services.

Second, stakeholders that we interviewed identified factors that encouraged the use of telehealth in Medicare, including the potential to improve or maintain quality of care, address provider shortages, and increase convenience to patients.

For example, telehealth can increase convenience by shortening or eliminating travel times, which may lead to better adherence to recommended treatment and to patient satisfaction. However, these stakeholders also identified several potential barriers to the use of telehealth in Medicare, including payment and coverage restrictions.

For example, officials from one provider association reported that Medicare's telehealth policies for payment and coverage, such as those restrictions that limit the geographic and practice settings in which beneficiaries may receive telehealth services, are more restrictive than the policies of other healthcare payers.

Finally, as of April 2017, CMS was supporting eight models and demonstrations that have the potential to expand the use of telehealth in Medicare. For example, one demonstration aims to develop and test new models of integrated healthcare in sparsely populated rural areas. Under the demonstration, CMS allows participating providers to receive cost-based payment for telehealth when their location serves as the originating site, rather than the approximately $25 fixed fee that CMS otherwise pays originating sites.

In summary, while the use of telehealth in select Federal programs is low, it remains an important alternative to providing healthcare services in person, especially for patients who cannot easily drive long distances for care.

Chairman, ranking members, and members of the Subcommittee, this concludes my prepared remarks. I would be pleased to answer questions at the appropriate time.

Chairman BLUM. Thank you Ms. Clowers.

I now recognize Ms. Johnston for 5 minutes.

STATEMENT OF BARB JOHNSTON

Ms. JOHNSTON. Thank you. Honorable Steve Chabot, Chairman Blum, and other members of the Subcommittee, my name is Barb Johnston as announced——

Chairman BLUM. Can you move closer to the microphone or move it closer to you? Thank you.

Ms. JOHNSTON. Does that work better? Okay. So sorry. I have been working in telemedicine for so long now I am thinking of lying. It has been over 20 years. It has been a labor of love. I have learned so much along the way. Today, I am here as a private citizen. I am doing that because I have been working in so many different areas, I wanted to cover lessons learned from so many of the opportunities I have had to work primarily serving people in rural areas.

As mentioned before, the core problem for rural medicine is 15 percent of the Americans who live there are only served by 10 percent of the Nation's doctors. Telemedicine has been around for a long time. Some of you may not know that psychiatry, telepsychiatry has been practiced for 50 years, half a century.

So far, there are some key things I wanted to share with you that have been demonstrated and that people have already mentioned, but I want to bring it up again. Telemedicine has shown and has massive capacity to keep rural dollars in rural communities. It supports rural primary care providers and clinics. It helps keep hospitals and clinics open. Without the support of specialists through these modalities that are so commonly used in our everyday life, such as using our cell phone, which is just a minicomputer or banking or education—people in this country expect to be able to use technology to receive appropriate and high-quality care using telemedicine, and it is happening. It is happening all over the country. It is growing.

It encourages recruitment and retention of the local doctors and providers who do serve physically in person in rural communities. Many, many studies, work that I have done, continues to show it does lower the overall cost of care. It can actually avoid small businesses closing. A person who owns a small business or a worker in a rural community who has to travel 3, 4 hours out site has to shut down that business that day. It costs them so much money and is so unnecessary. They lose wages, and the community may lose the barber shop, the only restaurant in town.

It also helps support health IT workforces. Every program I have ever started has included people in rural communities learning to use these technologies, and one thing you all should know: Rural people are very smart. They catch on very quickly. They are brilliant at putting these things together.

I think we all know that the cost of healthcare in this country is significant. It is growing. Telemedicine has the capacity to help resolve some of that financial burden. There are laws and regulations that could help significantly. I am identifying three that are crucial.

Number one is the problem we have with the DEA rule related to a 2008 bit of legislation called the Ryan Haight Act that inadvertently prevents our doctors providing the medication that they need so that when a telemedicine service is provided, specifically it affects three groups: Opiate addicts who need the medication, the doctors are not allowed to do the prescription online. All the doctors that we work with use electronic health records. They can't provide the drugs that these opiate addicts need. Our veterans, and I have seen a lot of them, they cannot receive the basic medications they need for PTSD, traumatic brain syndrome, just because of an inadvertent inclusion in that DEA rule. That could and should be changed and corrected. Children with ADDH, they lose school days. They can't pass because they can't get the medication they need.

One of the biggest problems we have had since Medicare instituted the rural requirement, this limits patients with Medicare who live in geographic locations that are defined by, in my opinion, very narrow rural designation; they can't receive Medicare services. Those constituents are getting more and more upset. They are seeing these things on TV. They know telemedicine exists. Medicaid doesn't have these rules, but Medicare does.

And the last one is the complicated credentialing licensing problems.

I see my time has run out. So I will leave where I am because I hit the key elements, and I am grateful, very honored to be allowed to present to you, and thank you so much for your consideration on this important topic.

Chairman BLUM. Thank you, Ms. Johnston. We are grateful that you are here, as well.

Mr. Adcock, you are recognized for 5 minutes for your testimony.

STATEMENT OF MICHAEL ADCOCK

Mr. ADCOCK. Thank you. Chairman Chabot, Chairman Blum, Ranking Members Schneider and Lawson, and members of the Small Business Committee, thank you for the opportunity to appear today. I am Michael Adcock, Executive Director for the Center for Telehealth at the University of Mississippi Medical Center in Jackson, Mississippi. I am honored to talk with you this morning about telehealth and the ways its power can be harnessed to address the healthcare needs of America's small businesses.

Mississippi has significant healthcare challenges, leading the Nation in heart disease, obesity, cardiovascular disease, and diabetes. These and other chronic conditions require consistent quality care, a task that is made harder by the rural nature of our State. In order to improve access to care and give Mississippians a better quality of life, it is clear that we need something more than traditional clinic and hospital-based services.

Telehealth has been a part of the healthcare landscape in Mississippi for over 13 years, beginning with an aggressive program to address mortality in rural emergency departments. This program has had a significant impact not only in bringing quality care to the residents of these communities but in supporting the viability of the community hospitals themselves. In some cases, TelEmergency prevented hospital closures that would have been detrimental to these underserved communities.

Today, the UMMC Center for Telehealth delivers care in over 200 sites in 68 of our State's 82 counties and provides access to patients who might otherwise go untreated. Maximizing our utilization of healthcare resources through the use of technology is the only way that we can reach all of the Mississippians who need care.

Small businesses account for 99.9 percent of all firms in the United States and often cite access to healthcare has their number one concern. Decreasing absenteeism, increasing productivity, and improving access to high-quality care are concerns to small businesses owners and were the drivers behind the creation of our eCorporate program at UMMC. This program allows employees to access high-quality care from their workplace through secure audiovisual connections, avoiding travel to seek medical care and promoting appropriate use of healthcare resources at a lower cost.

Several corporations have chosen to pay for this service for their employees and allow paid time during the workday to use the service, further reducing barriers to healthcare.

Should an employee have a need outside the scope of telehealth, UMMC assists in securing appropriate followup with local providers. The eCorporate program currently covers more than 4,000 employees and dependents statewide. We offer wellness services and diabetes prevention management services for corporations, as well.

Another program that has been very impactful for patients is remote patient monitoring, which supports patients as they manage these chronic diseases in their home. RPM is designed to educate, engage, and empower patients so they can take care of themselves. Our initial pilot with diabetics in the Mississippi Delta was a public-private partnership to test the effectiveness of remote patient monitoring using technology in rural, underserved areas.

The preliminary results showed a marked decrease in blood glucose, early recognition of diabetes-related eye disease, reduced travel to see specialists, and, most remarkably, no diabetes-related hospitalizations or emergency room visits among our patients.

The Mississippi Division of Medicaid extrapolated this data to show a potential savings of $180 million per year if 20 percent of the diabetics in Mississippi on Mississippi Medicaid participated in the program. Given the success of this diabetes pilot, UMMC Center for Telehealth has expanded remote patient monitoring statewide.

Healthcare is a major economic driver across the United States, and this has already been discussed. In Mississippi, hospitals boast over 60,000 full-time employees and create an additional 34,000 jobs outside of their facilities. For every new physician creates approximately 21 jobs and more than $2 million in revenue for our community. For every three jobs created by a hospital, an additional job is created by other businesses in the local economy.

Our telehealth program directly supports the financial viability of the healthcare system, especially primary care providers' offices, small rural hospitals, and rural healthcare clinics. Keeping services in the communities not only supports the local providers but keeps much needed employment and revenue in the rural communities.

Businesses in Mississippi that have utilized our telehealth and remote patient monitoring programs have seen improved access to care, decreased healthcare costs, and improved quality of care for their employees. Healthy employees mean decreased absenteeism, increased productivity, and a greater chance for small businesses to remain viable.

Thank you all for your time and attention to this very important matter.

Chairman BLUM. Thank you, Mr. Adcock.

And for some reason, you are a little easier to understand than my good colleague and friend, Mr. Kelly from Mississippi. So we appreciate that.

Dr. Schmitz, you are now recognized for 5 minutes.

STATEMENT OF DAVID SCHMITZ, M.D.

Dr. SCHMITZ. Good morning, Mr. Chairman, ranking members, and members of the Subcommittee. Thank you for inviting me here to testify. My name is David Schmitz, and I am a family physician who has practiced and taught in rural America for more than 20 years. I am here today representing the National Rural Health Association where I currently serve as president, and I am grateful to have this opportunity to discuss rural healthcare and its impact on rural America and local economies.

For 62 million Americans living in rural and remote communities, access to quality and affordable healthcare is a major concern. Rural Americans on average are older, sicker, and poorer than their urban counterparts, as we have heard. They are also more likely to suffer from chronic diseases that require ongoing monitoring and follow up care. Local care is necessary to ensure patient ability to adhere to the treatment plans to help reduce the overall cost of care and to improve patient outcomes and their quality of life.

Whether following the delivery of a healthy baby or significant loss of function due to stroke, local integrated care for rural people in their own support systems is not only the right care; it is better care.

Rural communities are resourceful, and the continuity of care is primary to good outcomes, such as avoidance of hospital readmissions. Investing dollars locally can save what would otherwise be wasted dollars lost to inefficiencies, anonymity, and the gaps that occur in the miles between.

There is no doubt that rural healthcare delivery is challenging. Workforce shortages, older and poorer patient populations, geographic barriers, low patient volumes, and high rates of publically insured Medicare and Medicaid recipients, uninsured and underinsured populations are just a few of the barriers.

Unfortunately, a growing number of rural Americans are living in areas with limited healthcare options. Indeed, 81 rural hospitals have closed since 2010, leaving many rural Americans without timely access to emergency care. Two of the most recent of these, closing on June 30 of this year, were in Florida and Texas.

As noted in my written testimony, health disparities between rural populations and their urban counterparts are pronounced, and this can be particularly true among the growing minority populations in rural America. Rural healthcare providers are not only critically important for health of rural Americans, they are also critically important for economic health of rural communities. While many industries in rural America have been shrinking, healthcare is an industry with the potential to reverse declining employment. As factory and farming jobs have declined, the local rural hospital often becomes the hub of the local business community, not only offering critical lifesaving services, but representing as much as 20 percent of the rural economy. Simply put, hospitals provide a large number of jobs.

The average critical access hospital creates 195 jobs, generates $8.4 million in payroll annually, and rural hospitals are often the largest or second largest employer in a rural community, along with the school system. This was true in the community I practiced in of 2,303 people for 6 years.

In addition, a single rural primary care physician, again as we heard, can generate as many as 23 jobs and more than a million dollars in annual wages, salaries, and benefits. In my own personal experience, rural communities are both resourceful and resilient. As referenced in my written testimony, training doctors and other health professionals close to home makes it more likely that they will call that place home.

In order for this to occur, we must have technology across a rural distributed campus, per se, training our workforce to meet the needs of rural communities and at the same time providing economic investment in those rural places.

Graduate medical education or residency training regulatory reform, allowing for education of physicians in rural hospitals, is one example of how to address rural economic development and workforce shortages in one action while improving quality of care and delivering cost-saving healthcare.

Technology. Technology, such as telemedicine for consultation services have supported rural delivery of care but depend on adequate development of broadband internet into rural and remote areas. Still hands-on care is needed when an unexpected car accident or early delivery of a premature baby occurs in rural America. No matter if you are a local resident or simply visiting, each one of us who will spend our time and dollars in rural communities, and at those times, will appreciate quality local care in those moments.

In addition to these lifesaving measures, healthcare is one industry capable of playing a critical role in supporting the local economy and protecting rural communities from further economic damage. If roads and internet access are the blood vessels and the nerves, then, in my opinion, healthcare is the backbone for investing in rural America.

Thank you again for the invitation to speak and to accompany my written testimony as submitted.

Chairman BLUM. Thank you, Dr. Schmitz.

I now yield to the chairman of the Subcommittee on Health and Technology, Ms. Radewagen, for her opening statement.

Chairwoman RADEWAGEN. Thank you, Mr. Chairman.

I want to apologize for being a little bit late. I was on the Senate side testifying on behalf of the Secretary Zinke's Assistant Secretary for Insular Areas, which is our areas.

So, talofa. Good morning. Thank you, Chairman Blum, and thank you all for testifying today. Good morning to Chairman Chabot, as well. It is an honor to chair the Subcommittee on Health and Technology, and I look forward to learning more today about how both health and technology can benefit small businesses and rural communities.

According to recent data from the Kaiser Family Foundation, American Samoa is facing tremendous shortages of primarily healthcare professionals and is currently only meeting around 10 percent of need in terms of the number of physicians available to serve the population. The Samoan Islands have among the highest rates of obesity and type 2 diabetes in the world, with one-third of American Samoans suffering from diabetes.

If medical treatment is unavailable on the island, patients, including many VA beneficiaries, generally have to fly nearly 3,000 miles to Hawaii to see a specialist. Recently CMS granted a waiver that will allow Medicaid patients to go to New Zealand instead. That has been helpful.

I am very interested in hearing and learning more about strategies for increasing the use of telehealth in rural and remote areas, like American Samoa, where provider shortages are severe. I also look forward to hearing more about how telehealth could attract more new or current physicians to locate their practices in rural areas, like American Samoa, where the tropical scenery, rain forests, beaches, and reefs are second to none.

I want to thank all the witnesses for being here today, and I yield back my time to Chairman Blum.

Chairman BLUM. Thank you, Ms. Radewagen, and thank you for that commercial at the end. We agree with you.

I now recognize myself for 5 minutes of questions. I love this topic. I think, you know, the increase in costs in healthcare in our country are not due to one large thing or two large things. I think, and pardon the pun, it is death by a thousand cuts. The increased costs are because of a thousand smaller things, and I also think the solution is not one silver bullet to solving increased access and decreased costs while keeping our quality high. There is not one silver bullet. I think it is a thousand smaller things, if you will. I absolutely believe one of those things smaller things is telemedicine.

I would like—this is for the whole panel—ideas of where—the Federal Government is the largest purchaser of healthcare in the country, obviously. I would like to hear from you places the Federal Government can increase the outcomes, the quality of the outcomes, increase access, decrease costs by utilizing telemedicine that we are not doing today. Give me two or three great examples of here's where we can save money and increase—improve the outcomes for patients. Anyone?

Dr. Schmitz.

Dr. SCHMITZ. Thank you, Mr. Chairman.

Just a couple of brief examples. One is you have heard the use of Tele-Emergency medicine. Again, how can you develop a relationship between a, for example, family physician and a critical access hospital; being able to be simultaneously supported both in their practice, which retains them, and also lowering the barrier to recruiting to rural areas. At the same time the transfer, if necessary, is expedited with high quality care.

Another example is tele-ICU or intensive care unit, consultation, allowing again, patients to stay in place, when possible. A third example is something called Project ECHO, which is a learning group where you can have essentially development of teams across the spectrum disease, including opioids, to be able to develop better practices across the country. And my final and fourth would be, again, the use of technology in telemedicine in distributed medical education and health professions education, training people as close to home as possible.

Chairman BLUM. So these items you just mentioned, Doctor, are not being done today?

Dr. SCHMITZ. To a certain extent they are, but there are also opportunities with regard to reimbursement mechanisms and regulatory mechanisms that would allow this to be expanded, particularly into rural areas. One example I mentioned was graduate medical education funding and residency funding reform, allowing again, more cost-based reimbursement or more support of these both workforce initiatives as well as healthcare delivery mechanisms.

Chairman BLUM. Thank you.
Are there others?
Ms. Johnston?

Ms. JOHNSTON. Thank you. I think the market has the potential to drive expansion massively if the handcuffs could come off, and I mean that in reference to my earlier remark, the limitation of the location of a patient being rural or not rural. It actually doesn't make any sense to me. It doesn't make sense to constituents when you have a neighbor who has Medicaid and they can see a doctor, and their next-door neighbor has Medicare and they can't, and that conversation is growing. I am hearing—I am an active member of the American Telemedicine Association, so I hear it from my colleagues all over the country. If that one thing could get corrected, I think the market would drive expansion, and it would help business in this country.

The other place is in skilled nursing facilities. Skilled nursing facilities primarily are caring for our elderly, some disabled, and in those facilities, almost all of the ones that we have approached even when I was in the position of having millions of dollars to fund programs, which I did, I couldn't get one nursing home to accept starting a program for fear that there would be an incorrect billing and they would be doing fraud, or because they would have some of their clients not being able to access care, and they didn't want to look like they were preferentiating one group over another.

Chairman BLUM. Mr. Adcock?

Mr. ADCOCK. Yeah, another area that is not currently being paid for through Medicare, not being reimbursed with Medicare, is remote patient monitoring, so chronic disease management in patients' homes. As we know, Medicare recipients often struggle from many chronic diseases, not just one, but diabetes, heart disease, and that is something we can impact through remote patient monitoring. Right now, there is not a payment mechanism for remote patient monitoring through Medicare.

Chairman BLUM. Do you feel this would actually save the government money or improve the outcome?

Mr. ADCOCK. Absolutely. Yes. I mean, similar to what we have done in Mississippi with Medicaid, I definitely—Medicaid, obviously, in Mississippi, is funded by Federal and State dollars. There is a tremendous savings just in diabetes. So, yes, we are performing this service in congestive heart failure, hypertension, asthma, COPD. There are many different chronic modalities that are costing a lot of money, and a lot of our healthcare resources that can be taken care of in the home through technology.

Chairman BLUM. Thank you.

And now my time has expired, and I now recognize the ranking member, Mr. Schneider, for 5 minutes.

Mr. SCHNEIDER. Thank you, Chairman Blum.

And thanks again to the witnesses for being here and sharing your perspective.

Ms. Johnston, I just want to say you should not be hiding the fact that you have been working this area for so long, but wearing it as a badge of honor because it is critical.

And I will also say you mentioned that we've been doing telehealth in psychiatry for 50 years. One of the things that struck me is that the phone was patented—and I had to look it up—the phone was patented in 1876. As we have new technologies, I don't want to wait 100 years or 90 years to start using them again.

Much of the conversation is often around telehealth filling gaps. If—for rural communities, there are gaps in care. Mr. Adcock, I think as you were talking about what you are doing in Mississippi, it's creating opportunities to improve healthcare, improve its efficiencies, lower its costs, and have better outcomes. And I hope, over the course of time, we can move our conversation from filling the gaps to really finding ways to use telehealth to make a difference. I think the rural communities and the small businesses, as you discussed, provide that great opportunity. So I will get off my soap box, but I did want to just emphasize that.

Dr. Schmitz, you said you've been in this area for a long time. We hear about the shortage of doctors for so long. Earlier this year, I was privileged to introduce the reauthorization of the Conrad 30 program, which would bring doctors from other countries into our rural communities helping to fill that gap again. But I would be curious from your experience, if you have seen that program and other programs of graduate medical education to support doctors coming into where the need is the greatest, share your thoughts, please.

Dr. SCHMITZ. Thank you, Ranking Member Schneider. I appreciate the opportunity to answer. We have seen benefits. There is no doubt about the need that we have, from a provider workforce standpoint, in rural America. And I think programs as such you have mentioned have been an important opportunity to be able to serve those needs.

I actually have done research looking at the recruitment of rural providers into both several States here in the United States as well as comparing that to other countries, such as in Australia, and I think as we look at a global need with regard to, as you said, not only beginning to have an adequate workforce in place, but really have a healthcare team that provides the most efficient and effective care to people, that the advent of technology has really changed the dynamic. Not only do we see doctors who still do house calls, but we also see physicians and really healthcare teams that can deliver everything from occupational therapy to dietician services and, most critically, mental health services locally as a team through use of technology and local providers. It is still about the relationship, isn't it, between the patient and the provider, between a couple of neighbors in a small town, that really I think to a certain extent impacts the quality of care and some of that efficiency, but supporting those providers as teammates and the use of technology has really changed the dynamic. And I think the example of health monitoring, where patients are empowered to be able to then access local healthcare and subspecialty care as needed, can change the fabric of what that appears to be. That will draw graduates from all over the world, I think, to appreciate what it means to be part of a rural community and a provider in those communities.

Mr. SCHNEIDER. Great. Thank you.

Mr. Adcock, you talked about your program, and I just want to clarify that I heard it right. Emergency diabetes check-ins went to zero in the program, you said?

Mr. ADCOCK. That is correct. The first—of the members of the study, they had zero ER visits, zero hospitalizations for the first 6 months of the program.

Mr. SCHNEIDER. That is extraordinary.

Mr. ADCOCK. It is.

Mr. SCHNEIDER. Are there things that you identify that were critical to that? Are there barriers to taking a program like this across the country?

Mr. ADCOCK. I think that the critical barrier—I mean, the critical success factors were the fact that we didn't just monitor. There are a lot of monitoring programs. Even though we call our program remote patient monitoring, we actually engage with the patient and provide them education. So I think providers—all the providers I have talked to would agree that, if they had the opportunity to educate their patients in small bits every single day and check on them and provide real-time intervention, they would, but that is not realistic.

So that is something we can deliver through technology. So that is where they benefitted was learning about their disease process. Diabetes, while it is not complicated to me or some of the providers, it is complicated to someone who is newly diagnosed and doesn't understand what they should eat, what they shouldn't eat, when they should exercise, how much water they should drink. So, when you can provide that education in a home daily in small, bite-sized pieces, it is extremely beneficial to them. And, also, when they slip or when they make a mistake and they eat the pecan pie, which we often do, when they check their blood sugar, we know it, and we are able to intervene immediately instead of waiting 3 months for the next in-person visit.

So I think it is that relationship and the engagement and the empowerment; teaching them to take care of themselves was the big success factor.

Mr. SCHNEIDER. Thank you.

And I am out of time. I just want to add one more comment. Ms. Clowers, thank you for the testimony, but the discussion around the different pilots that you all are doing to take those pilots where there are successes and getting it out, if there is anything we can do to help, please look to us.

And, with that, I yield back. Thank you.

Chairman BLUM. Thank you, Mr. Schneider.

And I will recognize the gentleman from Mississippi, Mr. Kelly, who is also our chairman of the Subcommittee on Investigations, Oversight, and Regulations for 5 minutes.

Mr. KELLY. Thank you, Mr. Chairman.

And, Mr. Adcock, it is nice to have someone here who does not have an accent.

Mr. ADCOCK. It took a lot of practice.

Mr. KELLY. How does Medicare's definition of rural area—and I know Ms. Johnston talked about this to—present challenge for providers wishing to incorporate telehealth into their practices, and specifically I know, in Union County, because one little area is so many miles from a four-way, they don't qualify, but from a four-lane highway, but people don't understand: Driving distance and miles are different, especially in rural areas. So, if you can do that, Ms. Johnston, after him, if you would like to follow up, I would really appreciate that.

Mr. ADCOCK. We talk a lot about rural versus urban settings and rural designations. What we see in telehealth, and Mississippi is certainly rural, and we have a lot of rural areas. We also have urban areas that don't qualify for as a CMS service. So I would like to steer the conversation away from geography. The fact is we have healthcare resource shortages, and it doesn't matter. I can tell you a specific example. Dermatology in Mississippi, it takes 6 months to get a dermatology appointment in Mississippi. It doesn't matter if you live right next to the University of Mississippi Medical Center or if you live 180 miles away. Geography doesn't matter in that case.

So it is more to me about healthcare resource shortages and being able to address those. Those don't always happen exactly the certain distance from a four-lane highway; they happen all over the place. So being able to lose that geographic restriction would be great, if we could lessen that or get rid of it all together, because the fact is access to care isn't just about urban versus rural. It is about whether or not there is a resource available and how a patient can access that resource.

Mr. KELLY. Ms. Johnston, briefly.

Ms. JOHNSTON. Thank you. Let me give you two quick examples. Number one, a small town in Wyoming where they have a huge backlog, patients needed to see a psychiatrist. They absolutely refused to allow us to provide telepsych, an entire program paid for, because they were so afraid of complications with not billing correctly. That is just one example.

Second example, we have been recently approached to provide telepsychiatry services to Puerto Rico. They identified six clinics. They gave us the addresses. We went online because there is a site under CMS to make sure that you are allowed to do it because they require that the Medicare also be seen. Not one clinic across Puerto Rico was considered to be meeting that definition. The program cannot go forward. I have been to Puerto Rico. I have driven all over it. I still can't find a nonrural area.

Mr. KELLY. And that being said, you know, Mr. Adcock, I want to ask this question, but I think it is important: It is more economy driven than it is rural or urban. There are a lot of inner city areas that have the exact same issues that rural areas have. They have the exact same travel distance or challenges that a rural area would have, and I think it becomes about people who are a lot of times impoverished, who don't eat well, and who are not educated in what those diseases are, and are a long distance in time or access from medical, and I think we owe it to them to get medical access and I think telehealth can do that. That being said, Mr. Adcock, what are the benefits of small businesses offering telehealth in the workplace?

Mr. ADCOCK. I think, again, it is access. It allows access for employees who may not have access to healthcare otherwise. Also, it forms that relationship. Once they start seeing a provider, and we are able to refer them to a local primary care physician, it completes that relationship. And the earlier they can get access to care, the more likely they are to recognize a disease, whether it be prediabetes, whether it is diabetes, hypertension, it could be, you know, eye disease, any other disease. So early access is important. And limiting those barriers.

So a lot of employees are main providers for their home. They are not able to take off half day to go to a physician's office, and they may have to drive 40, 50 miles to the physician's office, wait in the waiting room, be seen, and they have missed half a day of work, they have to pay their copay, they will just be sick. And employees who aren't well aren't productive. It is not good for the small business. So being able to decrease absenteeism, increase productivity is extremely important for those small businesses and could mean the difference between keeping them viable or not.

Mr. KELLY. And just in closing, Mr. Chairman, I will just say telehealth is the wave of the future. We know preventative medicine is one of the primary cost-saving benefits that we get in America, and using technology to get that is a no-brainer to make sure that we use this and maximize this for small businesses and for our medical care.

Thank you, and I yield back.

Chairman BLUM. Well said. Thank you, Mr. Kelly.

And I now recognize the gentleman from Florida, Mr. Lawson, who is also the ranking member on the Subcommittee on Health and Technology for 5 minutes.

Mr. LAWSON. Thank you.

Dr. Schmitz, rural America includes approximately 57 million people and about 20 percent of the population. There are 1,855 rural hospitals that support nearly 2 million jobs. How does improved access to care in rural areas benefit the local economy?

Dr. SCHMITZ. Thank you, Congressman.

You are exactly right that, again, the testimony that I provided in writing and accompanying here with you is that local hospitals are a driver of the local economy, not only directly with regard to employment of physicians that results in economic stimulus and further jobs, but also, with regard to keeping the opportunity for growing other businesses local.

Again, I have had experience in North Dakota but also now 20 years of experience in Idaho, and I can remember times when, during difficult fiscal discussions, we talked about roads and we talked about healthcare and we talked about education because we knew that would bring industry to our small towns. That was an economic driver in itself but also built, again, a framework upon which we could see economic growth.

So I would commend the opportunity to speak with you and agree on the fact that rural hospitals, and at this point, in particular in time, saving rural hospitals, recognizing not only their cost effectiveness to quality care but also the fact that they are an economic driver in our Nation is a timely discuss. Thank you.

Mr. LAWSON. Okay. Thank you.

And, Doctor, I am going to ask you this question simply because I was involved in it. In 2000, we in the legislature in Florida authorized a medical school at Florida State, and a key factor in authorizing that medical school is that they were going to train physicians to go into rural areas because other people might want to comment on that. So that has been 17 years later, but what I understand, and a lot of these students once they finish, because of tremendous loans and stuff in medical school, they want to go into the cities where they can make a little bit more money to take care of medical loans. Have you seen in medical schools, has this philosophy changed, and have we worked out anything to cause them to go into rural areas?

Dr. SCHMITZ. Thank you, Congressman. That has been the study of my last 10 or 15 years since leaving rural practice myself but staying in contact with rural medicine as a medical educator. I think you are right that we have found that intentional public accountability with regard to medical education is key, and training in interprofessional health teams is also important.

One of the things that I have seen is that we train to have people remain. I could say being from the country from the sticks, training in the sticks' sticks. And one of the things that we have found is that, with studies we have actually done, including rural training track residency education, where we actually have physicians training during their residency in rural places such as critical access hospitals have a higher likelihood that those physicians will remain in rural and underserved communities.

So I think those sorts of investments and the opportunities to look at regulatory relief or funding and then encouraging again our medical schools to have these sorts of tracks for rural providers shows that there is the evidence, is that, where they train, they are more likely to remain. This accompanied by loan repayment opportunities, both at the Federal and State level, and mentoring—frankly, mentoring of physicians, so that they can see themselves there, especially now in the advent of the utilization of technology where now we can see our patients are supported to be self-empowered around their disease conditions. But, frankly, I think that I can tell you, as a 29-year-old doctor in an ER, it is a little bit scary, and you want to do the best you can, and you know you will do the best you can, but having an opportunity to have that consultation and mentoring, not only in person and in practice with your partners but also through telehealth, makes a powerful statement to our young students.

Mr. LAWSON. My time has almost expired, but, Ms. Johnston, since you have been at it for a very long time, do you see any difference of it really working in the training in medical schools, a physician to go right in the rural areas?

Ms. JOHNSTON. I think one of the strategies that we have done in the State of California, I served on the board of trustees for the

Health Education Foundation, and what that sought to do, and it has been very effective, we provide loan repayment for primarily physicians but other healthcare workers who will serve in rural areas. That has been the most successful thing we have ever done, because some of these students get out, they owe $150,000, and to get them to go work in a rural area where their income is going to be so much lower than in the urban area, this was a huge incentive. And it has been a very effective program. And we found that, if they stay in the rural community for 2, 3, 4, 5 years, much higher percent that they will stay there.

Mr. LAWSON. Okay.

And I yield back, Mr. Chairman.

Chairman BLUM. Ms. Clowers, did you want to add on to that quickly?

Ms. CLOWERS. Thank you. I just wanted to add that we did work issued early this spring where we looked at graduate medical education funding, and most of the funding is still going to urban areas, and that is important, as Dr. Schmitz said, because where people train, they tend to stay. And also what we found is that the Federal efforts to increase graduate medical education in rural areas is limited, and really that funding is driven by statute. So I just wanted to add that for the Subcommittee.

Chairman BLUM. Thank you.

Thank you, Mr. Lawson.

The gentleman from Kentucky, Mr. Comer, is recognized for 5 minutes.

Mr. COMER. Thank you, Mr. Chairman.

I have a question for anyone on the panel. Just out of curiosity. I assume you all kept track of both the House healthcare bill and the Senate healthcare bill. And I am curious, did either of those bills affect telehealth in any way either positively negatively or no impact whatsoever? Anybody know?

Mr. ADCOCK. I don't have any idea.

Ms. JOHNSTON. No.

Mr. COMER. What about a complete repeal? That is something that is obviously being batted around now in the Senate and in the House. Would a complete repeal have any impact on telehealth, a complete repeal? Anybody know?

Ms. JOHNSTON. I can only imagine that, if millions of Americans lose their health insurance, it is going to have an impact on this Nation. And it for sure is going to impact anywhere healthcare is provided.

Mr. COMER. But there is no specific part that you can think of that would have a—I mean, you just assume that?

Ms. JOHNSTON. I would agree with that. Probably the best source to get that specific answer would be through the American Telemedicine Association. They have staff that are specifically looking at this. And we can follow up and get that information to you from the ATA.

Mr. COMER. I certainly support telehealth. Being in a rural part of Kentucky, it is very challenging for our hospitals to get physicians. And this is very important. And we want to certainly support that. And, hopefully, we can work together and fix our broken healthcare system. There are parts of healthcare that are working.

There are parts that I think need to be radically changed. The cost of healthcare is a big issue that doesn't seem to be getting a lot of attention now. It is all about health insurance. But, hopefully, we can come to a solution and look forward to staying in contact with you all as we try to fix our broken healthcare system. And, certainly, for those of us that represent rural areas, telehealth is a very, very important part that I want to support, and I am sure everyone on this Subcommittee does as well.

Thank you, Mr. Chairman.

Chairman BLUM. Thank you, Mr. Comer.

The gentleman from Kansas, Dr. Marshall, is now recognized for 5 minutes.

Mr. MARSHALL. Thank you so much, Mr. Chairman. A great topic, something I am pretty familiar with.

I think, first of all, always talking about success stories. Colby, Kansas, Citizens Hospital. Part of the stroke collaborative program that Dr. Bobby Moser has piloted in Kansas, one of the greatest success stories I have ever seen, very dependent upon telemedicine. A person has an acute onset of a stroke. And if we can get that thrombolytic agent within 30 minutes—we talked about cost savings, so much about cost savings. The true cost savings that this makes is in the healthcare dollars that we are not going to spend. This stroke person that we prevented this stroke from becoming permanent, we just have saved hundreds of thousands of dollars of hospital bills, rehabilitation bills, and then a person that is maybe on a disability the rest of their life.

So that is the beauty of this. We could talk about strokes. We could talk about acute MIs, again, using that thrombolytic agent. And what people don't understand is these agents have very significant side effects. And it takes a lot of courage to give this drug. And if you don't give it on a regular basis, you just don't give it, especially not in time. The nurses drag their feet. So Colby, Kansas, is hooked up 24/7 to another busy, busy ER, and a nurse can take the patient's symptoms. And while the nurse practitioner is scrambling to get over there, walks into the room, and everything is already set up and going. They have got a protocol set. We are getting the CAT Scan, and within 30 minutes, we can give that drug. And it is night and day.

Another great success story in Kansas is the Kansas Enhanced Veterans Service Program. It is a mobile office that goes across the State. Twenty-two veterans die from suicide every day in this country. Those veterans are not going to come to the veterans hospital, both of them, that we have in Kansas. So we are taking the program to them. They are using telemedicine to touch base with their psychiatrist, their psychologist, their social workers back home, making sure they get their medicines. Absolutely a success story.

My thoughts would be is that government will not solve this problem but, rather, innovation will continue to solve the problem. And Medicaid or Medicare is typically in the way of solving the problem. So I just would just continue to look for success stories and then try to, not reinvent the wheel, but keep accentuating those.

So I would ask for anyone, what are the most—I shared my success stories. We can't use a shotgun and try to use telemedicine for everything. But it has some great opportunities in the emergency room, and I think the psychology/psychiatry as well.

So does anyone have a great success story they want to share? Dr. Schmitz, you have one?

Dr. SCHMITZ. Thank you, Congressman. Again, I would just share a success story around tele-ICU. And what that is, essentially, is in, again, a critical access hospital that otherwise can provide appropriate care—I have certainly been in a situation where we were, frankly, weathered in. We were concerned about the safety of having a helicopter land in our town because of snow or other conditions, also similarly concerned, what would a patient be able to do with regard to ground transport for safety? In my town, there were 104 curves in a 19-mile piece of road on the way out to the urban center. So I think you are exactly right.

And one thing we can look at is, how do we have consultation through telemedicine with, for example, patients who may or may need to be transferred the next morning and oftentimes actually don't need to be transferred? Again, providing not only quality care, access to care, but in a fairly common scenario better care, and likely empower that team.

Mr. MARSHALL. I have been in that same position so many times with a 25-week baby, 600-gram baby, fogged in, snowed in, and scrambling to try to fix that problem. I can certainly deliver that baby, but the problem was taking care of the baby afterwards.

Any other great success stories that you have?

Ms. Johnston, go ahead.

Ms. JOHNSTON. I was PI on the Patient-Centered Medical Home Project. That was a program funded through CMS' CMMI innovation initiative. And during the 2 years—3 years that we ran it, 2012 to 2015, we showed significant cost effectiveness. Just as one example, NIH, their numbers for outpatient for mental health patients annually averages about $1,557. Ours came out to $390. Patient satisfaction, over 90 percent. It was huge.

Mr. MARSHALL. So I got 20 seconds. Where is telemedicine not working? Can you give me examples, anybody, where there is an area of medicine that it hasn't worked very well?

Ms. JOHNSTON. No.

Mr. MARSHALL. Yes, sir.

Dr. SCHMITZ. I do think we need to continue to coordinate care so patients have primary care access, and electronic medical records that are able to integrate patients' global care.

Mr. MARSHALL. Thank you.

Chairman BLUM. Thank you, Dr. Marshall.

The gentleman from Nebraska, Mr. Bacon, is now recognized for 5 minutes.

Mr. BACON. Thank you very much to all four of you. We have got votes coming up. So I will just get right to the questions. I appreciate you being here.

First of all, a couple of you mentioned the definition for rural areas hurt telehealth. Is that a regulation or a law? What do we need to change, specifically, to fix this?

Ms. CLOWERS. For Medicare, it is defined by statute.

Mr. BACON. Okay. So it is on us to make that change then?

Ms. CLOWERS. Correct.

Mr. BACON. Okay.

Ms. CLOWERS. And what it requires is, it requires both in terms of restrictions on the facilities as well as the location. So certain facilities are allowed, in Medicare, to be an originating site.

Mr. BACON. Right.

Ms. CLOWERS. As well as, it has to be located in an area that has been defined by HHS as being a health professional shortage area or outside of a metropolitan area.

Mr. BACON. So that is a task for us to work on then. We will take that on.

Second question, Ms. Clowers, you mentioned the VA using a lot more telehealth. Can you talk a little more about that? Because I know we have a big long line of people trying to get care, and this is one way to help.

Ms. CLOWERS. Right. VA, what we found is that 12 percent of beneficiaries in 2016 were provided telehealth visits, which is much greater than what we saw in Medicare. And, in fact, what we also found was that they have over 50 different types of specialties or services that are eligible for telehealth, and they have less restrictions than in Medicare. So, for example, the program does allow for the patient to be at home for telehealth visits.

Mr. BACON. That is great news.

Here is one for any of you all. Who are the opponents to doing this? Are there industries out there or institutions that are fighting us? Go ahead. Please.

Ms. JOHNSTON. I think the world of telemedicine has appropriately been challenged by a lot of really important agencies, the American Medical Association used to be really concerned. I think the concerns all stem from people wanting to make sure that we are doing this correctly, that we are providing quality care. Whenever we get challenged, it is never from somebody who is just saying no. It is just because they need to be educated and reassured that anybody who's using these technologies is meeting, if not exceeding, the quality of care that people deserve.

Mr. BACON. One last question. It seems that some illnesses are tailor-made for this, but others may be a little more challenging. So what is the percentage, would you say, roughly, that this is—telehealth is perfect for? But there is other things—sometimes you got to lay eyes on the infection or—you know what I am saying? There are some things a little more challenging that the doctor has to actually see it, perhaps, or take blood or something. I don't know. What do you think the percentages are?

Dr. SCHMITZ. Congressman, thank you for that important question.

I think, first of all—and I think in response to the other question about the pending decisions that will come up around healthcare and access is in that rural America, we need to have people who can deliver healthcare and places where it can be delivered. So we look at rural health clinics, federally qualified health centers, private practices, and critical access hospitals as examples. We still need the providers there. If it is an automobile accident and a chest tube is required for a collapsed lung, we still need the providers there. I see telemedicine more to support those services, as well as to augment them.

And in some ways, telepsychiatry mental health, we have even seen where patients will be more likely to see a telehealth provider in an adjunct room of the critical access hospital as opposed to sometimes driving down the street a block. I don't know what the future holds. But I don't see one necessarily replacing the other. They really come together.

Mr. BACON. Well, thank you very much.

I yield back.

Chairman BLUM. Thank you, Mr. Bacon.

As has been mentioned previously, votes have been called. So this is a very important topic. And we have some members here that still haven't had a chance to ask their questions. So we will stand in recess until after the votes, and then we will reconvene.

We shall stand in recess.

[Recess.]

Mr. LUETKEMEYER. [Presiding.] Okay. We will gavel our Committee back into session. And thank all of the witnesses for continuing to stick around. I apologize for the delay, but we did have to do a little bit of what we are here to do a while ago, which is go vote on some very important legislation to certain people, areas of our country.

I am Congressman Luetkemeyer. I am from Missouri. I am the vice chair of the entire Committee. And Chairman Blum has other duties to attend to for the moment. So you are stuck with me to take us out the gate here.

So, with that, let us continue on with the discussion we are having, and we will recognize Miss González for 5 minutes.

Miss GONZÁLEZ-COLÓN. Thank you, Mr. Chairman.

And thank you, the whole panel, for staying here so long.

Over the last 5 years, over 3,000 physicians have left Puerto Rico. And, currently, the island loses one doctor per day, as you may know. Hospitals and medical practice groups are finding it very difficult to recruit specialist physicians and experts. We are trying to have some kind of telehealth by medical specialists located in the U.S.-based academy medical centers, maybe can be a great opportunity for the island, especially in rural areas that are a hundred percent of the island, maybe 90 percent. Are there any impediments to telehealth payment arrangement when the patient is located at their home in Puerto Rico or at a medical facility in Puerto Rico and the doctor is located at a medical center located on the mainland? Ms. Johnston?

Ms. JOHNSTON. Hi. It is Barb Johnston. Many. And it is problematic. As I mentioned, we have been approached, the company I currently work for. We have the doctors. They want to work. They have doctors locally that want to learn how to do this locally in Puerto Rico. And we are more than happy to do it. The sticking point is getting payment for doing it. As I said before, Medicare's rule that restricts to their definition of rural for telemedicine completely blows the whole project. It prevents us from being able to do that. If there could be some kind of a waiver, or if we could be allowed to pilot, or whoever is going to be able to provide the care—because it won't just be telepsych, which is what we do. There are others. But that is the desperate need that we have heard from people in Puerto Rico. So if they could do that.

The other is getting a waiver to allow patients to be seen in their home. There are many parts of Puerto Rico where—and we have been told—that people don't have transportation. Even if there was some, they can't. And, like, the Veterans Administration in this country has been doing this for 10 years successfully, seeing patients directly at home.

Miss GONZÁLEZ-COLÓN. Quick question. That waiver, it is going to be for the Federal Government or Federal—do we have to amend any Federal laws, or we are talking about State laws?

Ms. JOHNSTON. I might——

Miss GONZÁLEZ-COLÓN. I defer to Ms. Clowers.

Ms. CLOWERS. The requirement is through statute. So the statute defines in Medicare where the services can be provided. And as Ms. Johnston said, it has to be—the originating site must be in an area that has been designated as a health professional shortage area or outside of a metropolitan area.

Miss GONZÁLEZ-COLÓN. In our case, I mean, the shortage is there. Actually, we are having the same problems in the VA facilities, the same as the American Samoa, where we don't even have the specialists in so many areas in the VA hospital. And we have tried to recruit them, but it is so difficult. Because nobody wants to leave the mainland to go to Puerto Rico or even remote areas to just move their families to attend the patients there. And I would like to know if you can provide, the whole panel, specifically what kind of amendments do we need to make to change that statute? If you can provide—I mean, I know that we—in 1 minute, you can't provide that. But if you can provide that to the Committee later on, that will help us a lot to identify those statutes with the correct language so we don't mess—mess with the whole situation.

Ms. CLOWERS. And, Representative, I would like to add, too, that in addition to a potential statute change, CMS, through their innovation center, has different models and demonstrations that they can run. And they have the ability to waive certain requirements. And so they would have the ability to have a demonstration and waive these rural requirements.

Miss GONZÁLEZ-COLÓN. I know.

Ms. CLOWERS. If that would be something that you would be interested——

Miss GONZÁLEZ-COLÓN. I know. We are working with them directly and we are trying to change the State plan. And even doing that, we are still facing the same problems. That is happening in Puerto Rico. That is happening in other States. So this is not an issue just for—but we are facing—in our case, in the islands, you can't cross the State line. You can't take a car or even take a train. You have to take a plane or a boat to take the service, and that is not enough. So that was the question. Since my time is running, is there any—can you provide any information about the security of the patients' records on telehealth or how secure and private these records are when telehealth is employed?

Ms. JOHNSTON. The way that most of us work—and I will speak to the company I currently work for. We use a fully HIPAA-compliant system end to end. We use a product called athenahealth. I have no investment in it, don't own it. It is just a completely secure and HIPAA-compliant system. Anything that we use technologywise, the videoconferencing, the health records, any communication—you can't text. There is very strict—we actually are the only telepsych company in the country that is Joint Commission accredited. That is just part of it. But, yeah, end to end.

Mr. ADCOCK. Same thing. Ours is encrypted and all HIPAA compliant. Everything that we use goes into our electronic medical record, Epic. So it is all controlled just as it would be if you came in person.

Miss GONZÁLEZ-COLÓN. Thank you.
I yield back. Thank you, Mr. Chairman.
Mr. LUETKEMEYER. The gentlelady's time has expired.
Next we go to Representative Radewagen, from American Samoa. She is the Chairman of the Subcommittee on Health and Technology. You are recognized for 5 minutes.

Chairwoman RADEWAGEN. Thank you, Mr. Chairman.
Ms. Clowers, American Samoa could greatly benefit from using health for patients to access medical care remotely without leaving the islands. We talked about it a bit today. However, broadband access is not sufficient. Are there Federal programs available to assist remote areas like American Samoa to support broadband for telehealth?

Ms. CLOWERS. Yes, ma'am, there are. And you are correct, broadband is a challenge, and it is something that we heard in our work when we surveyed people about the barriers to using telehealth, the infrastructure that is required to successfully carry out telehealth. Broadband was identified as one of those infrastructure challenges. And there are grants that are available for different communities through different departments.

And, for example, the USDA has grants. And American Samoa has received a grant, I believe in the amount of $820,000, for support in this area. And we would be happy to get you more information on that grant, if you are interested.

Chairwoman RADEWAGEN. Thank you.
Mr. Adcock, what are some important innovations in telehealth that you have experienced while working in this field? And what innovations may we expect in the future as more American consumers demand telehealth services?

Mr. ADCOCK. Thank you very much. I think the innovations that we—I am going to go to the second part of the question first. The innovations that are coming in the future, I couldn't begin to tell you. There are so many different wearables and sensors and things that are coming out now, that are being innovated now, that I can't imagine what the future is going to look like from that standpoint.

But I think where we focus on technology is that we wrap technology around our clinical programs. I think that our focus—while technology is certainly important, I think our focus is around the patient and what we need to do to provide excellent clinical care to the patients, and then we use the appropriate technology around that. But being able to deliver care into a home to monitor diabetes so that patients don't have to plug anything in or try to transcribe their outcomes or their results themselves, I think that, just in the last couple of years, has come so very far. And being able to Bluetooth into these devices and use cellular technology to connect to patients and providers has come so very far in the last couple of years. Where it is going, I would honestly be scared to say. But I think that the focus needs to remain on making sure that providers and patients, not necessarily in that order, but patients and providers are the center of what we are doing with telehealth. This should be an extension of healthcare. This should be something that is used to help better healthcare services that can be delivered at home.

Ms. Johnston, would you care to answer that question?

Ms. JOHNSTON. I completely agree. At the American Telemedicine Association annual conference this last year, Thomas Friedman spoke, keynote, and that is really what he was echoing. He stood on a stage and said: Right now, with 10,000 people in this audience, there is a couple of guys in a garage in Silicon Valley, and they are ahead of us. We just need to catch up with them.

I think it is going to be part of it.

I think, too, the current president of the American Telemedicine Association, he has been putting forward and doing a lot of speaking about hybrid healthcare in a model that he sees more and more individual providers and health systems where they see some patients on telemedicine, use remote monitoring, and some in person. And that is happening quite a bit. It is spreading across major hospitals and health systems across the country. Thank you.

Mr. Chairman, I yield back.

Chairman LEUTKEMEYER. I understand the lady from Samoa has a closing statement. You can go ahead and do that.

Chairwoman RADEWAGEN. Thank you, Mr. Chairman.

Well, let me take this opportunity to thank all of the witnesses for their testimony today. As the chairman of the Subcommittee on Health and Technology, it is extremely valuable to hear how telehealth is helping physicians expand the services they offer and is offering patients more convenient options to access the healthcare they need.

American Samoa is facing tremendous provider shortages, and telehealth services could keep our residents and their families from traveling long distances to receive care or going without the care they need. This could also benefit other small businesses by keeping dollars in the community. I was also pleased to learn that there is hope that telehealth will make rural areas more viable locations for physicians to operate their practices. Technology has improved many aspects of daily life, and it can potentially improve healthcare access as well.

[Speaking foreign language.]

Thank you. And I yield back to Chairman Luetkemeyer.

Mr. LUETKEMEYER. I am glad you interpreted that for us. Thank you very much.

I will defer my questions to the end. I think Miss González has got a second round question here.

So let's go to Miss González. You are recognized for 5 minutes.

Miss GONZÁLEZ-COLÓN. Thank you, Mr. Chairman. I really appreciate that deference. I will be short. I will just leave you with some questions I got.

And one is regarding Mr. Kelly, in his statement here, identified the issues regarding rural areas. And one of the concerns regarding

Mississippi was the diabetes situation. And your experience treating patients with diabetes and using telehealth, how do they—those patients were improving. Do you have seen a decrease in the hospitalizations and emergency room visits in Mississippi? That is one of the questions, because we got the same situation in the island, and other situations regarding heart diseases, among others. That would be one of the questions. I don't want to abuse from the chairman. That will be one of the questions.

The second one is going to be in terms of is there a need for a certification requirement when telehealth providers are located in a jurisdiction other than where the medical provider is located? What of those requirements, if they are from a CMS, or HHS, or whatever they are, if the State is involved in that, and how difficult are those regulations to comply with? And in terms of having—is there any copayment to the patient if they are using health in terms of the veterans, if they are using this kind of program? I don't know. That is going to be one of the questions.

Mr. ADCOCK. I will take the first question around remote patient monitoring. And thank you for asking that followup question. Yes. In our diabetes pilot that we did in the Mississippi Delta, we saw significant results in the preliminary results. And the final results will be out later this month. But we saw a decrease in hemoglobin A1c, which is the measurement of blood sugar over time. We also saw a complete elimination of ER visits and hospitalizations for those patients that were on our program. So, not only did they just reduce their visits to the ER, we did not have any diabetes-related ER visits or hospitalizations.

Miss GONZALEZ-COLON. Zero?

Mr. ADCOCK. Zero. Not saying that that would be sustained over a huge population. But we have seen very similar results in our—the final results are very much mirroring that. And the results that we see with our population that is on that program outside of the pilot have had significant results in readmissions and hospitalizations. So that is one of the points of the program. But I think the reasons for that are because of the education that we provide and the real-time interventions. So we teach them about their disease so that they can take care of the disease themselves. You can't expect them to go to a provider every time something is going on. That is not realistic. It is not realistic for the provider. It is not realistic for the patient. So being able to teach them about their disease and then teach them as they are having issues so, if their blood sugar goes up, you are able to intervene at that time and say: This is why your blood sugar went up. This is what you can do to prevent it in the future. A lot of these ER visits aren't due to medical emergencies every time. A lot of times they are due to fear. They don't know what to do when this happens. So being able to educate them in real time has been a real success. And we have spread that program statewide.

Miss GONZALEZ-COLON. Mr. Schmitz.

Dr. SCHMITZ. Thank you, Congresswoman. I would just like to agree with that testimony and just give a quick example. If we look, for example, as a primary care provider, a family physician, per se, at the patient-centered medical home having a dashboard where information comes in, you can literally have, you know, green, yellow, red where people who are knowledgeable about this data can then, for example, use what is called open-access scheduling and decide who gets an acute care visit open slot with that provider, be it a physician assistant, physician, or otherwise, and avoid, again, that lack of information that otherwise might result in an ER encounter with someone who does not know them as well.

Miss GONZÁLEZ-COLÓN. Thank you.

Ms. Johnston or Ms. Clowers?

Ms. CLOWERS. To your second question about other challenges with licensing, when we spoke to different stakeholders through our work, we did hear that licensing was a challenge. And an example of that is when you are at the distant site—if you are a provider at the distant site, you also have to be licensed in the State that the patient resides. And that can be challenging for different providers. And that is driven by State law.

Miss GONZÁLEZ-COLÓN. Thank you. You want to add something, Ms. Johnston?

Ms. JOHNSTON. I was just going to answer—I think you asked a question about a copayment for telemedicine?

Miss GONZÁLEZ-COLÓN. Yes. Is there——

Ms. JOHNSTON. I have never actually heard of that. I don't have any experience with that.

Miss GONZÁLEZ-COLÓN. Okay.

Ms. JOHNSTON. We have never done anything like that.

Miss GONZÁLEZ-COLÓN. Okay. Thank you.

With that, I will yield back.

Thank you, Mr. Chairman.

And thank you, all the members of the panel.

Mr. LUETKEMEYER. The Gentlelady's time has expired.

With that, I just want to follow up with a few things.

And I know that, Ms. Clowers, you were talking about some of the payment and coverage restrictions that cause problems sometimes. I think it was Ms. Johnston mentioned some of the things that happened and can be done or changed with regards to the locations qualifying. But with regards to payment and coverage restrictions, can CMS do this right now through their rulemaking process, or does that take legislation?

Ms. CLOWERS. The coverage issue would require legislation. It is defined by statute.

Mr. LUETKEMEYER. Okay.

Ms. CLOWERS. They do have flexibilities in their innovations center where they are able to test different approaches with different models and demonstrations. So that would be an area that they could explore with a model.

Mr. LUETKEMEYER. Okay. Some of the things you talked about, do you have studies that show how much it saves?

Ms. CLOWERS. We do not. When we did our work in looking at the different opportunities, both benefits of telehealth, we were looking at CBO scores which showed—it is hard to tell sometimes in terms of the cost savings. It depends on how telehealth is used. If it is used to replace an in-person visit, that can result in savings. But if it is used in addition to an in-person visit, that can increase cost. So that is what we found in terms of the cost savings. But I know other witnesses here at the table have other experiences.

Mr. LUETKEMEYER. Yeah. I think, Mr. Adcock, you were talking about your in-home monitoring programs. And did you put an analysis on that and see how much you actually saved with the pilot project you are talking about?

Mr. ADCOCK. So the pilot project, again, was a public/private partnership. But our division of Medicaid actually took the data on the actual cost savings of those first 100 patients, first 6 months, and extrapolated that to say that, if 20 percent of the Medicaid patients in Mississippi who were diabetic were on the program, we would save $180 million a year. So, yes, there are cost——

Mr. LUETKEMEYER. Your State would save that much?

Mr. ADCOCK. Yes. Yes. Medicaid would save that much so federal and state together—

Mr. LUETKEMEYER. The State Medicaid program would save $180 million——

Mr. ADCOCK. Correct.

Mr. LUETKEMEYER.—a year just on that one——

Mr. ADCOCK. Just diabetics, just 20 percent. So now we are doing hypertension and heart failure and all the other chronic diseases we are monitoring as well. So we will continue to do cost analysis on those programs. We have legislation in Mississippi that allows us to get paid for remote patient monitoring. So there is a fee to it, and we do receive payment. The cost savings are tremendous.

Mr. LUETKEMEYER. Okay. And you mentioned a couple other things that you are working on with your more remote abilities here. And that was heart monitoring and what else?

Mr. ADCOCK. Heart failure. So congestive heart failure. Hypertension. That is adult and pediatric diabetes. We are working on asthma and chronic obstructive pulmonary disease. All of these are high-cost items. We also monitor—this is outside of the reimbursement legislation in Mississippi. We also monitor bone marrow transplant and kidney transplant patients so that we can get them out of the hospital sooner and get them back home.

Mr. LUETKEMEYER. The hearing today was with regards to rural telehealth. But, I mean, telehealth is something that they can utilize—people can utilize every day everywhere else too, many urban areas, suburban areas. I mean, this isn't something confined. But what we are talking about here is the importance of how it helps the quality of life, basically, for folks in rural areas.

And so, Dr. Schmitz, would you like to add anything to the discussion with regards to other opportunities and the cost savings? Have you done any studies or are aware of any of that?

Dr. SCHMITZ. I really appreciate the opportunity, Congressman. One example, I think, that hasn't been brought up is the provision of chemotherapy, for example. As you can imagine, in a rural critical access hospital that is quite remote from subspecialty care, supporting a local physician/nurse team, for example, to administer chemotherapy in the same quality really does prevent patients who otherwise would have very uncomfortable transport—not only long transport, but uncomfortable transport, during the treatment of their disease.

Mr. LUETKEMEYER. Okay. So what we are doing is trying to find ways to improve the quality of health and health services in rural areas. And the things you are suggesting, is anybody putting this into a bill that you are aware of or just discussed it with you to help work on this?

Yes, sir, Dr. Schmitz.

Dr. SCHMITZ. I would be happy to follow up with National Rural Health Association how telemedicine and teletechnologies can be incorporated into better care——

Mr. LUETKEMEYER. Because the comment a minute ago was that some of it has to be done legislatively; some of it can be done through the rulemaking process. I think we have a friend with Dr. Price at HHS now who is willing to look at options, look at different things, different ways to deliver care, deliver services, upgrade and innovate. But by the same token, if we need to do something legislatively, I think that is where we need to go.

Mr. Adcock.

Mr. ADCOCK. The CONNECT for Health Act that is out right now addresses a lot of these issues.

Mr. LUETKEMEYER. Okay.

Mr. ADCOCK. It addresses the geography issues, addresses a lot of the reimbursement issues. So that is something that we fully support and would love to see some more input on that.

Mr. LUETKEMEYER. Very good.

Yeah. Ms. Johnston?

Ms. JOHNSTON. I just want to second that that legislation is bipartisan, the CONNECT for Health. It would address most of these things.

Another comment I would like to make, in the CMS grant that we were given, 2012-2015, we submitted a final report that showed significant cost savings. Happy to provide that to the Committee. The VA every year produces very good data on cost savings. And the American Telemedicine Association is currently collating data on multiple studies across the country on cost savings.

Mr. LUETKEMEYER. Does the VA coordinate with—I guess it is CMS with regards to telehealth stuff? I mean, your veterans are scattered all over the place. I mean, and they network back, usually, to a VA facility of some sort. Does that help them or hurt them with access to care? Are you familiar with that?

Ms. JOHNSTON. I don't know that the VA works in any capacity with CMS. But I know that they are the largest provider of telemedicine in this country and have been. Nobody is even close to what they have been doing, and they keep proving every year how cost effective it is every year for our veterans.

Mr. LUETKEMEYER. Okay. Very good. I am at the end of my questions. Would you all just like to have a closing question or comment or go ahead and say goodbye? Tired of listening to us?

Yeah. Dr. Schmitz.

Dr. SCHMITZ. Congressman, I would be just happy to first be the one to say thank you for the opportunity to speak about the important matters in rural health. I do think that we are seeing technology both to change access as well as quality of care and as we continue to see this again, as our panelists discussed, as a wraparound, person-to-person services, I think we will have better care for it. The example with the VA, for example, CBOCs, and how CBOCs can actually be co-located with other provider of services and co-supported through technology might just be one more example. So, again, Congressman, thank you for this opportunity.

Mr. LUETKEMEYER. Mr. Adcock.

Mr. ADCOCK. I would like to echo that. Thank you for the opportunity to come and talk about this important subject. Thank you for your interest and your very thoughtful questions. I do think that telemedicine is a way that we can spread access and improve quality across not just the United States but across the world, certainly across everything that the United States encompasses. So I think that is extremely important. And I thank you for your questions and for the time to speak.

Mr. LUETKEMEYER. It is also great to know not everybody in Mississippi talks like Mr. Kelly.

Ms. Johnston, closing comment?

Ms. JOHNSTON. I just want to echo what has been said. But also just from myself thank you for what you do every day for Americans.

Mr. LUETKEMEYER. Thank you.

Ms. Clowers.

Ms. CLOWERS. Thank you for having us. And at GAO, we are happy to stand ready to help with any further discussions on this topic.

Mr. LUETKEMEYER. Very good.

With that, again, I want to thank everybody for being here. As we heard, telehealth has the ability to connect a patient in a rural area to high-quality medical care at another location. This not only benefits the patients and their families but also may help the local physician to expand his or her small business. Other small businesses will benefit from dollars staying in the community. Additionally, we have heard that the availability of telehealth may attract new or current physicians to locate practices in rural communities and also how telehealth can benefit small employers and employees by offering convenient access to medical care and monitoring. In fact, I would think it would be an attractive way to attract doctors to the rural area if they know they can do it with telehealth and be—the quality of life is—coming from a town of 300 people—it is a whole lot better than it is in the city. So, therefore, why not move to the country, right? But with consumer demand growing for more convenient and efficient options to access healthcare, I hope that we are able to sort out some of the barriers our witnesses have testified about so that small businesses and rural communities have all the tools they need to thrive and keep residents well.

Well, with that, I ask unanimous consent that members have 5 legislative days to submit statements and supporting materials for the record.

Without objection, so ordered.

We are adjourned.

[Whereupon, at 12:34 p.m., the Subcommittees were adjourned.]

APPENDIX

GAO

United States Government Accountability Office

Testimony

Before the Subcommittee on Agriculture, Energy, and Trade and Subcommittee on Health and Technology, Committee on Small Business, House of Representatives

For Release on Delivery
Expected at 10:00 a.m. ET
Thursday, July 20, 2017

TELEHEALTH

Use in Medicare and Medicaid

Statement of A. Nicole Clowers, Managing Director, Health Care

GAO Highlights

Highlights of GAO-17-760T, a testimony before the Subcommittee on Agriculture, Energy, and Trade and Subcommittee on Health and Technology, Committee on Small Business, U.S. House of Representatives.

July 2017

TELEHEALTH

Use in Medicare and Medicaid

Why GAO Did This Study

Telehealth can provide an alternative to health care provided in person at a physician's office, particularly for patients who cannot easily travel long distances for care. Medicare pays for some telehealth services that are subject to statutory and regulatory requirements, such as requiring the patient be present at an originating site like a rural health clinic.

This testimony discusses (1) the extent to which telehealth is used by Medicare and Medicaid to provide health care services; (2) factors selected associations representing providers, patients, and payers reported as affecting the use of telehealth in Medicare; and (3) how emerging payment and delivery models could affect the potential use of telehealth in Medicare.

This testimony is based on GAO's April 2017 report (GAO-17-365). For that report, GAO reviewed agency documents and regulations and interviewed Medicare agency officials and Medicaid officials from six states, selected based on multiple factors, including rural population. GAO also selected specialty associations with expertise and interest in telehealth—five provider, two patient, and one payer association—based on a review of documents and literature and through background interviews. GAO interviewed representatives from each of the associations and also collected information from the provider and patient associations through a data collection instrument. In addition, GAO reviewed agency documents describing and evaluating the models and demonstrations that support alternative approaches to health care payment and delivery.

View GAO-17-760T. For more information, contact A. Nicole Clowers at (202) 512-7114 or clowersa@gao.gov.

What GAO Found

Available analysis GAO reviewed shows that Medicare providers used telehealth services (providing clinical care remotely by 2-way video) for a small proportion of beneficiaries and relatively few services in calendar year 2014. Specifically, an analysis of Medicare claims data by the Medicare Payment Advisory Commission shows that about 68,000 Medicare beneficiaries—0.2 percent of Medicare Part B fee-for-service beneficiaries—accessed services using telehealth. The most common telehealth visits in calendar year 2014 were for evaluation and management services (66 percent), followed by psychiatric visits (19 percent). In Medicaid, the use of telehealth varies by state. Individual states have the option to determine whether to cover telehealth, what types of telehealth services to cover, and which types of providers can receive reimbursement for telehealth services, among other things. In the six states GAO reviewed, officials from states that were generally more rural than urban said they used telehealth more frequently than officials from more urban states.

Selected provider, patient, and payer associations GAO interviewed reported that telehealth may improve care for Medicare beneficiaries, but they also cited coverage and payment restrictions as barriers to the use of telehealth in Medicare.

- Officials from the selected associations reported several factors that encourage the use of telehealth in Medicare, including the potential to improve or maintain quality of care in Medicare, alleviate provider shortages, and increase convenience to patients. For example, officials from one provider association noted that provider and regional medical specialty shortages can be addressed through telehealth, potentially increasing productivity and ensuring on-time scheduling of appointments.
- Officials from the selected associations also reported several potential barriers to the use of telehealth in Medicare, including payment, coverage restrictions, and infrastructure requirements. For example, officials from one provider association and both of the selected patient associations described access to sufficiently reliable broadband internet service as a barrier to telehealth use.

The Centers for Medicare & Medicaid Services (CMS), which administers Medicare, has various efforts underway that have the potential to expand the use of telehealth in Medicare. As of April 2017, CMS was supporting eight such models and demonstrations. For example, CMS's Frontier Community Health Integration Project Demonstration aims to develop and test new models of integrated health care in sparsely populated rural counties. Under the demonstration, CMS allows participating providers to receive cost-based payments for telehealth when their location serves as the originating site, rather than the approximately $25 fixed fee that CMS otherwise pays originating sites.

_____ United States Government Accountability Office

Chairmen Blum and Radewagen, Ranking Members Schneider and Lawson, and Members of the Subcommittees:

I am pleased to be here today to discuss the use of telehealth in Medicare and Medicaid.[1] For certain individuals, such as those who live in remote areas or who cannot easily travel long distances, access to health care services can be challenging. Telehealth can provide an alternative to health care provided in person at a physician's office by providing clinical care remotely through two-way video for services such as psychotherapy or the evaluation and management of conditions. Medicare pays for some telehealth services subject to statutory and regulatory requirements, such as the requirement that the patient be present at a site such as a rural health clinic. Telehealth services in Medicaid may vary from those provided in Medicare, as individual states determine whether to cover telehealth services and any requirements for such coverage. At the federal level, the Centers for Medicare & Medicaid Services (CMS), an agency within the Department of Health and Human Services (HHS), administers Medicare and is responsible for overseeing state Medicaid programs.

My testimony today summarizes the findings from our April 2017 report on telehealth.[2] Accordingly, my testimony addresses

(1) the extent to which telehealth is used by Medicare and Medicaid to provide health care services;

(2) factors that selected associations representing providers, patients, and payers reported as affecting the use of telehealth in Medicare; and

(3) how emerging payment and delivery models could affect the potential use of telehealth in Medicare.

To conduct the work upon which this statement is based, we reviewed agency documents and regulations and interviewed Medicare agency officials and state Medicaid officials from six selected states—Connecticut, Illinois, Kansas, Mississippi, Montana, and Oregon—which

---

[1] For this testimony, we define telehealth as clinical services that are provided remotely via telecommunications technologies.

[2] GAO, *Health Care: Telehealth and Remote Patient Monitoring Use in Medicare and Selected Federal Programs*, GAO-17-365 (Washington, D.C.: April 14, 2017).

we selected based on variation in geography, physical size, percentage of rural population, and other factors related to coverage and reimbursement for health care services. We also obtained documents from and interviewed association officials from general and medical specialty associations with expertise and interest in telehealth—five provider, two patient, and one payer association—which we selected based on a review of relevant documents and literature and through background interviews. We also collected information from the provider and patient associations through a data collection instrument. In addition, we reviewed CMS documents describing and evaluating models and demonstrations that support alternative approaches to health care payment and delivery. More detailed information on our objectives, scope, and methodology for that work can be found in the issued report. We conducted the work on which this testimony is based in accordance with generally accepted government auditing standards. Those standards require that we plan and perform the audit to obtain sufficient, appropriate evidence to provide a reasonable basis for our findings and conclusions based on our audit objectives. We believe that the evidence obtained provides a reasonable basis for our findings and conclusions based on our audit objectives.

Use of Telehealth in Medicare and Medicaid

As we reported in April 2017, available data from the Medicare Payment Advisory Commission (MedPAC) show that Medicare providers used telehealth services for a small proportion of beneficiaries and relatively few services in calendar year 2014, the latest data available at the time of our audit work. In Medicaid, the use of telehealth varies by state.

Medicare

Medicare pays for certain telehealth services, including consultations, office visits, and office psychiatry services.[3] While telehealth visits with providers are conducted from a separate site, Medicare requires that the patient be physically present at a medical facility such as a hospital, rural health clinic, or skilled nursing facility—referred to as the originating site—

---

[3]Medicare payment for telehealth services in Medicare fee-for-service is limited to those on CMS's approved list of telehealth services. Plans within Medicare Advantage—the Medicare managed care program—must cover the same telehealth services as those provided through fee-for-service, though Medicare Advantage plans can provide additional telehealth benefits not on CMS's approved list to their beneficiaries by using rebate dollars or charging beneficiaries a supplemental premium. Plans must receive CMS approval in order to provide the additional telehealth benefits.

during the telehealth service.[4] Eligible providers who are furnishing Medicare telehealth services are located at a separate site, known as the distant site, and these providers submit claims in the service area where their distant site is located.[5] The originating site is paid a facility fee—about $25 in calendar year 2017—under the Medicare Physician Fee Schedule for each telehealth service, and the distant site provider is paid the same rate for services delivered via telehealth as they would be paid for the in-person service, as required by statute.[6] (See fig. 1.)

---

[4]By statute, originating sites are limited to those located in rural health professional shortage areas, counties not included in a metropolitan statistical area, and sites participating in a federal telehealth demonstration project (referred to as telemedicine demonstration projects in statute) approved by or receiving funding from the Secretary of Health and Human Services as of December 31, 2000. Eligible originating sites are a physician or provider office, a critical access hospital, a rural health clinic, a federally qualified health center, a hospital, a hospital-based or critical access hospital-based renal dialysis center or satellites, a skilled nursing facility, and a community mental health center. 42 U.S.C. § 1395m(m).

[5]Eligible telehealth providers in Medicare are physicians, physician assistants, nurse practitioners, clinical nurse specialists, certified registered nurse anesthetists, nurse-midwives, clinical social workers, clinical psychologists, and registered dietitians or nutrition professionals.

[6]Medicare pays for physician and other health professional services based on a list of services and their payment rates, called the Physician Fee Schedule.

Figure 1: Example of Telehealth Use in Medicare

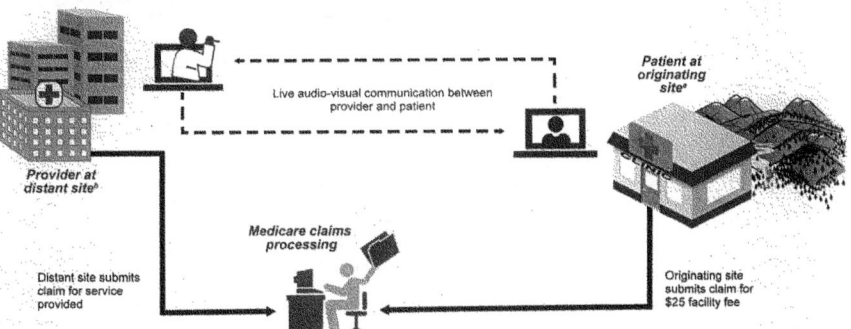

Source: GAO analysis of Medicare statute and regulations. | GAO-17-760T

[a] Medicare requires that the patient be physically present at a medical facility—referred to as the originating site—such as a hospital, rural health clinic, or skilled nursing facility during the telehealth service.

[b] Eligible providers who are furnishing Medicare telehealth services are located at a separate site, known as the distant site.

In April 2017 we reported that available calendar year 2014 data show that Medicare providers used telehealth services for a small proportion of beneficiaries and relatively few services. An analysis of Medicare claims data by MedPAC shows that about 68,000 Medicare beneficiaries—0.2 percent of Medicare Part B fee-for-service beneficiaries—accessed services using telehealth.[7] According to MedPAC, beneficiaries accessing telehealth averaged about three telehealth visits per person per year in calendar year 2014, and Medicare spent an average of $182 per beneficiary, for a total of about $14 million. MedPAC's analysis shows that 10 states accounted for 42 percent of all Medicare telehealth visits, with South Dakota, followed by Iowa and North Dakota, accounting for the highest use—more than 20 telehealth services were provided per 1,000

---

[7] See Medicare Payment Advisory Commission, *Report to the Congress: Medicare and the Health Care Delivery System*, (Washington, D.C.: June 15, 2016), 229-260. Part B services include physician and outpatient hospital services.

fee-for-service beneficiaries.[8] The most common telehealth visits in calendar year 2014 were for evaluation and management services (66 percent), followed by psychiatric visits (19 percent). MedPAC reported that physicians and nurse practitioners were the most common providers participating in telehealth visits in calendar year 2014 and, of all providers, behavioral health clinicians, including psychiatrists, made up 62 percent of providers at distant sites.

Medicaid

In our April 2017 report we found that CMS does not limit the use of telehealth in Medicaid; therefore, individual states have the option to determine whether to cover telehealth, which types of telehealth services to cover, and which types of providers can receive reimbursement for telehealth services, among other things. We interviewed Medicaid officials from six selected states and among these officials, the ones from states that were generally more rural than urban said they used telehealth more frequently than officials from more urban states. For example,

- Montana officials told us they have used telehealth as a tool to help patients see both in-state and out-of-state specialists remotely, as there is limited access to specialists in the state. According to state officials, Montana's Medicaid spending on telehealth increased from the state's fiscal years 2013 through 2015. Specifically, according to officials, Montana's Medicaid program spent about $132,194 for 1,841 distant site claims related to telehealth in fiscal year 2013, and this amount increased to about $284,675 for 3,218 such claims provided in fiscal year 2015.

- In contrast, officials from Illinois, which contains more urban areas, told us that telehealth represented a very small portion of the state's overall Medicaid budget and was used primarily to provide psychiatric services. According to state officials, less than $500,000 of Illinois' $20 billion in Medicaid spending in state fiscal year 2015 was for telehealth.

---

[8]The other seven states are—in rank order of use of telehealth per 1,000 beneficiaries—Wyoming, Nebraska, Minnesota, Missouri, Montana, Texas, and Oklahoma.

Selected Associations Reported That Telehealth May Improve Care for Medicare Beneficiaries but Cited Coverage and Payment Restrictions as Barriers

Our April 2017 report found that officials from selected provider, patient, and payer associations reported several factors that encourage the use of telehealth in Medicare, including the potential to improve or maintain quality of care in Medicare, alleviate provider shortages, and increase convenience to patients. For example, officials from one provider association noted that provider and regional medical specialty shortages can be addressed through telehealth, potentially increasing productivity and ensuring on-time scheduling of appointments. Officials from another provider association reported that telehealth can increase convenience by shortening or eliminating travel times—which may lead to better adherence to recommended treatments and to patient satisfaction.

Officials from the selected provider, patient, and payer associations also reported several potential barriers to the use of telehealth in Medicare, including payment and coverage restrictions. For example, officials from one provider association reported that Medicare's telehealth policies for payment and coverage—such as those restrictions that limit the geographic and practice settings in which beneficiaries may receive telehealth services—are more restrictive than the policies of other health care payers. Additionally, officials from the selected associations reported infrastructure requirements as another barrier to the use of telehealth in Medicare. For example, officials from one provider association and both of the patient associations described access to sufficiently reliable broadband internet service as a barrier to telehealth use.

CMS Has Various Efforts Underway That Have the Potential to Expand the Use of Telehealth in Medicare

Our report found that as of April 2017, CMS was supporting eight models and demonstrations that have the potential to expand the use of telehealth in Medicare. In these models and demonstrations, CMS has waived certain Medicare telehealth requirements or restrictions, such as requirements for the locations and facility types where beneficiaries can receive telehealth services. For example, the waivers allow beneficiaries receiving care under the models or demonstrations to access telehealth in urban areas or from their homes.

In another example, CMS is supporting a demonstration that could increase the amount a facility is paid when it serves as the originating site. CMS's Frontier Community Health Integration Project Demonstration aims to develop and test new models of integrated health care in sparsely populated rural counties. Under the demonstration, CMS allows participating providers to receive cost-based payments for telehealth when their location serves as the originating site, rather than the approximately $25 fixed fee that CMS otherwise pays originating sites.[9] CMS officials told us that as of January 2017, they did not have data on the utilization of the originating site facility fee waiver, as the demonstration had only been operational for a few months.

Chairmen Blum and Radewagen, Ranking Members Schneider and Lawson, and Members of the Subcommittees, I would be pleased to answer any questions that you may have at this time.

GAO Contact and Staff Acknowledgments

If you or your staff members have any questions concerning this testimony, please contact me at (202) 512-7114 or clowersa@gao.gov. Contact points for our Offices of Congressional Relations and Public Affairs may be found on the last page of this statement. Other individuals who made key contributions to the statement include Carolyn Yocom (Director), Karen Doran (Assistant Director), Sarah Resavy (Analyst-in-Charge), Krister Friday, and Helen Sauer. Staff who made key contributions to the report upon which this statement is based are identified in that report.

---

[9] The Frontier Community Health Integration Project Demonstration had 10 rural health care participants, and of those, 8 had telehealth as a demonstration intervention tool.

This is a work of the U.S. government and is not subject to copyright protection in the United States. The published product may be reproduced and distributed in its entirety without further permission from GAO. However, because this work may contain copyrighted images or other material, permission from the copyright holder may be necessary if you wish to reproduce this material separately.

GAO's Mission	The Government Accountability Office, the audit, evaluation, and investigative arm of Congress, exists to support Congress in meeting its constitutional responsibilities and to help improve the performance and accountability of the federal government for the American people. GAO examines the use of public funds; evaluates federal programs and policies; and provides analyses, recommendations, and other assistance to help Congress make informed oversight, policy, and funding decisions. GAO's commitment to good government is reflected in its core values of accountability, integrity, and reliability.
Obtaining Copies of GAO Reports and Testimony	The fastest and easiest way to obtain copies of GAO documents at no cost is through GAO's website (http://www.gao.gov). Each weekday afternoon, GAO posts on its website newly released reports, testimony, and correspondence. To have GAO e-mail you a list of newly posted products, go to http://www.gao.gov and select "E-mail Updates."
Order by Phone	The price of each GAO publication reflects GAO's actual cost of production and distribution and depends on the number of pages in the publication and whether the publication is printed in color or black and white. Pricing and ordering information is posted on GAO's website, http://www.gao.gov/ordering.htm.
	Place orders by calling (202) 512-6000, toll free (866) 801-7077, or TDD (202) 512-2537.
	Orders may be paid for using American Express, Discover Card, MasterCard, Visa, check, or money order. Call for additional information.
Connect with GAO	Connect with GAO on Facebook, Flickr, LinkedIn, Twitter, and YouTube. Subscribe to our RSS Feeds or E-mail Updates. Listen to our Podcasts. Visit GAO on the web at www.gao.gov and read The Watchblog.
To Report Fraud, Waste, and Abuse in Federal Programs	Contact: Website: http://www.gao.gov/fraudnet/fraudnet.htm E-mail: fraudnet@gao.gov Automated answering system: (800) 424-5454 or (202) 512-7470
Congressional Relations	Katherine Siggerud, Managing Director, siggerudk@gao.gov, (202) 512-4400, U.S. Government Accountability Office, 441 G Street NW, Room 7125, Washington, DC 20548
Public Affairs	Chuck Young, Managing Director, youngc1@gao.gov, (202) 512-4800 U.S. Government Accountability Office, 441 G Street NW, Room 7149 Washington, DC 20548
Strategic Planning and External Liaison	James-Christian Blockwood, Managing Director, spel@gao.gov, (202) 512-4707 U.S. Government Accountability Office, 441 G Street NW, Room 7814, Washington, DC 20548

Please Print on Recycled Paper.

Congress of the United States

U.S. House of Representatives
Committee on Small Business: Subcommittees on Agriculture, Energy, and Trade and Technology

21ˢᵗ Century Medicine: How Telemedicine Can Help Rural Communities

July 20, 2017

Testimony of Barb Johnston, MSN, ML&M
CEO, HealthLinkNow, Sacramento, California
Fellow, American Telemedicine Association

Honorable Steve Chabot, Chairman and other Members of the Subcommittee:

I am Barb Johnston, testifying as a private citizen who has been working in Telemedicine for many years including more recently as a Co-Founder and CEO of a small business Telepsychiatry company. Prior to this I was Executive Director of the Medical Board of California. I am a former Board Member of the American Telemedicine Association where I am also a Fellow. I have served since 2006 as a Founding and current Board Member of the California Emerging Technology Fund whose mission is to deploy broadband to rural and underserved communities across California. Having worked in Telemedicine since 1995, I offer these comments as lessons learned from the public we serve, healthcare providers, regulatory bodies, government agencies, and colleagues in our industry. Although my comments are meant to focus on the economic effect of Telemedicine in rural communities, many of these remarks will also relate to non-rural environments.

The core problem in rural medicine is that the 15% of Americans who live in rural areas are serviced by only 10% of the nation's physicians. To maintain and improve the Economic Vitality of Rural America it is essential that rural people are kept healthy and that rural communities are supported by a full range of medical services, delivered both in person, and increasingly, by telemedicine.

Telemedicine has demonstrated its effectiveness over the past 50 years and already benefits Rural America by:
a.   Keeping <u>rural dollars in rural communities</u>, and providing access to much needed and more timely Healthcare services
b.   Supporting Rural Primary Care providers and clinics and ensuring local health facilities, including hospitals, remain open
c.   Encouraging the recruitment and retention of local physicians and other healthcare providers who can be supported by telemedicine providers
d.   <u>Lowering the overall costs of care</u> and avoiding unnecessary ambulance transportations, emergency visits and hospitalizations
e.   <u>Avoiding small businesses closing down</u> each day that an owner or worker has to travel for healthcare, and also preventing rural people losing work days because they have to travel for healthcare

f.   Supporting health IT workforce development for rural healthcare workers

Economic Impact of Telemedicine
The potential economic impact of widespread implementation of TM across Rural America will be significant and holds promise to create a more efficient and effective healthcare system, lower overall costs and improve economic vitality of Rural America.

"According to statistics from the Organization for Economic Cooperation and Development (OECD), the United States spends more on health care than any other OECD nation, both in absolute terms and as a percentage of gross domestic product (GDP). In 2015, the United States spent $9,450 per capita on healthcare, representing 16.9% of GDP. That represents an inflation-adjusted increase of nearly 23% since 2005.₁ Forecasts show these expenditures continuing to grow.[1] The Centers for Medicare & Medicaid Services, for example, forecasts total U.S. health expenditures to grow by 5.6% per year between 2016 and 2025, and to outpace GDP growth by 1.2% per year over that period." [2]

TM has been expanding in both urban and rural America and patients have begun asking for this convenience. People, especially rural people, can't afford to drive hundreds of miles to urban clinics, losing wages and paying for eating out if appropriate care can be provided via TM in their own community. There are over 200 TM identified networks in the United States. More hospitals and health systems are implementing TM services to improve access to care, lower healthcare costs, recruit and retain providers and more and more people are expecting the benefits of TM. Americans use their computers (cellphones/laptops/desktops) for everyday life: education, banking, shopping, news, and communications and they now expect to access some healthcare services via TM.

Brian Whitacre, an associate professor and extension economist in the department of Agricultural Economics at Oklahoma State University, researched TM travel cost and lost wages (for rural Arkansas, Kansas, Oklahoma, and Texas) and projected annual travel costs savings based on mileage from $2,303 to $109,080 with a mean of $24,210. He estimated annual lost wages between $4,188 to $68,269 and a mean of $19,761. Dollars not spent on unnecessary travel can stay in rural communities. Rural America can simply not afford to lose wages when TM could prevent it.

Telemedicine Laws and regulations needed to support Rural America
With changes to regulations and laws as suggested below specific high demand telemedicine services will be possible, and will lead to extra clinical and economic benefits accruing to rural communities.

---

[1] Schadelbauer, Rick, "Anticipating Economic Returns of Rural Telehealth
NTCA-The Rural Broadband Association, March 2017 (1).

[2] Centers for Medicare & Medicaid, National Expenditures Projections, 2016-2025
https://www.cms.gov/Research-Statistics-Data-and-Systems/Statistics-Trends-and-Reports/Natioanl/HealthExpenddata/Downloads/proj2016.pdf

The changes I recommend are;

1. **Modify DEA rules to allow physicians to prescribe controlled substances by telemedicine.** This will benefit the following 3 specific sets of patients who need treatment with controlled substances that cannot currently be prescribed by telemedicine.
    i. Opiate Addicts who need medication assisted treatment,
    ii. Veterans with PTSD and TBI, and
    iii. Children with ADHD

2. **Change the CMS rural rule to enable Medicare patients despite geographic location to receive telemedicine services.** This will open up more rural telemedicine services, especially for seniors in nursing homes.

3. **Simplify national credentialing and state reciprocal medical licensing processes to enable telemedicine psychiatric and specialist medical services to be increasingly linked into rural primary care clinics.** This will give rural communities better access to medical experts.

The following are details of my recommendations:

I. **Change the DEA rules to allow physicians to prescribe controlled substances for patients who receive their care via telemedicine.** This will especially benefit the following 3 specific sets of patients who need treatment with controlled substances that cannot currently be prescribed by telemedicine.
   - Opiate Addicts who need medication assisted treatment,
   - Veterans with PTSD and Traumatic Brain Injury (TBI), and
   - Children with ADHD

The DEA has not followed through on required rulemaking regarding the **Ryan Haight Act** of 2008 which inadvertently affected the TM industry making it impractical to prescribe controlled substances by TM. Although DEA was meant to make this correction in October 2015 it has not and has no announced plans to modify the Act. The three groups of patients most adversely affected by this ruling are prevalent in rural regions, are of great political sensitivity and importance, and lack of treatment for all leads to considerable costs, both clinical and economic. The continuing inability to properly treat these patients adversely impacts rural economic vitality in a major way. These patients are forced to travel to urban centers for care or to suffer with lack of care.

I recommend that either Congress or the DEA should make emergency rules to allow providers to prescribe controlled substances, as recommended by the American Telemedicine Association, at least initially for mental health and psychiatric services, including addiction treatment.

II. **Change the CMS rural rule to enable Medicare patients despite geographic location to receive telemedicine services.** This will open up more rural telemedicine services, especially for seniors in nursing homes. Medicare's narrow definition of rural as relates to reimbursement of healthcare provided via TM prevents most Medicare beneficiaries from access to healthcare via TM. Medicaid does not have this "rural" limitation. Medicare constituents should have the same benefits that Medicaid constituents enjoy.

Changing this rule is especially important for patients in Skilled Nursing Facilities (SNF), primarily seniors with some rehabilitation and disabled patients. As Executive Director of the California Telemedicine and eHealth Center (CTEC) 2003-2007, I travelled across urban and rural California to fund Telemedicine (TM) programs primarily targeting underserved communities. Despite efforts to fund skilled nursing facilities not one SNF determined to accept the funds or assistance to pilot TM. As Principle Director of the CMS funded Patient-Centered Medical Home for Mental Health program 2012-2015 SNF patients were able to access much needed Telepsychiatry services. Unfortunately after that award funding ended the program could not continue in large part because of the Medicare rural rule. What I found was:

- Rural SNFs have a severe lack of access to specialists including but not limited to psychiatrists, dermatologist, cardiologists, etc. Patients are commonly behaviorally disturbed and at times receive excessive amounts of tranquillizers except when reviewed by psychiatrists and geriatricians, both of which are in very limited supply in-person in rural communities.
- Studies have shown that SNF patients do clinically much better when reviewed by psychiatrists and/or geriatricians, are less sedated, have less medications and have less expensive transfers out of the SNF
- Most SNFs do not meet the "rural rule" for Medicare reimbursement and therefore are not able to use Telemedicine so that patients can access health services via TM.
- Because CMS will not reimburse for TM unless the location is in a narrowly defined "rural" location many health facilities refuse any TM programs because of concern over billing problems, being perceived as providing preferential services to the non-Medicare patients.
- **Medicare is the only health insurance payor who limits access to healthcare via TM related to geography.**
- Rural SNF's have difficulty recruiting and retaining General Practitioners (GP). TM can provide a vehicle for a GP, and other specialists, to support an onsite Nurse Practitioner at the SNF.
- Physician shortages can lead to closure of a SNF which can lead to local unemployment, and the move of patients to other regions away from their families.
- The implementation of TM usually relies on existing staff, upskills those staff and frequently leads to job satisfaction and employee retention.
- Lack of specialists available for a SNF, such as psychiatrists, requires patients to be transferred usually by ambulance to a hospital many miles away to then be held in an emergency department for several days waiting for a psychiatrist or other specialist to evaluate the patient. This scenario is cost prohibitive and usually involves payment from either Medicare of Medicaid. Costs include the ambulance each way, the emergency department stay and the specialist. The rural SNF also loses revenue each day the patient is away and they cannot "give away" the patient's bed. Because the specialist is so far away, the patient may require follow up ambulance transportations to and from the emergency department or

- clinic office with the loss to local rural economy growing and bills to CMS escalating.
- Even if a physician begins a practice in a rural community where he/she has a solo practice which requires 365/days a year and 24/7 call coverage it usually can't last long. Time off, let alone vacations, become difficult to impossible. This work load inevitably leads to burnout or losing that one provider. Support from telemedicine providers is known to markedly improve in-person physician retention.

III. **Telemedicine should be routinely integrated into Rural Primary Care:** CMS through its Center for Medicare Medicaid Innovation (CMMI) Initiative awarded $7.7million to a small business Telepsychiatry company between 2012 and 2015 to develop and implement a new model of care where a Telepsychiatry network was integrated into over 80 Primary Care clinics across Wyoming, Montana and Washington State. Patients were followed up after their psychiatric consultations by virtual care navigators who checked on medication and lab work compliance. The goals were to prove this model would improve access to health care, assure patient satisfaction and reduce the per capita cost of care. These goals were achieved. Patient satisfaction data collected by an independent third party reported that the 96% of patients who had received care via this Telepsychiatry program would recommend Telepsychiatry to friends and family and **81% preferred Telepsychiatry to in person** psychiatry. Significant cost savings were also achieved.

Poor adherence to medication regime for patients suffering mental illness often leads to a choice between suicide, homicide, drugs/alcohol, poverty, and emergency department visits/hospitalizations. Adherence to medication was monitored for the schizophrenic patients in this program at 99% which is extremely high. Patients with all other mental illnesses (depression, anxiety, bipolar, etc.) in our project had a 96% adherence to medication regime. Key factors to this outcome included the fact that patients received care in the clinics they normally went to-their rural primary care (PCP) doctor's office. Stigma was reduced as no one knew they were seeking mental health care via their PCP. Patients and families didn't have to drive miles away with the cost of gas and eating out so money stayed locally and less time was lost from work.

Key findings of the cost effectiveness of this Telepsychiatry model of care as reported to CMS include the following;

- NIH reported in 2006 that the average cost of outpatient mental health for adults was $1,551/year and for children $1,931. Mental illness accounts for $193B in lost earnings per year. (http://www.nimh.nih.gov/health/statistics/cost/mental-healthcare-cost-data-for-all-americans-2006.shtml)
- Over 50% of US counties have no psychiatrist and psychiatrists practicing now are retiring in large numbers with no one to replace them.
- In this Telepsychiatry integrated into Primary Care model the average costs of care was $390/patient/year. Patients were seen by a psychiatrist via TM, who made a diagnosis and developed a treatment plan which were given directly to the patient and their own PCP in their rural community. In most cases the patients were able

to be followed by their PCP since the Telepsychiatrists had established the diagnosis and the treatment plan.

IV. **Regulatory barriers to the entire Telemedicine Industry**
   1. **Credentialing** requirements delay onboarding physicians both in person and as TM providers. Credentialing requires massive amounts of information to assure physicians are in good standing and qualified. Credentialing in itself is appropriate but the problem is that every health facility requires the physician to be credentialed over and over again. Each credentialing process takes between 2 to 6 months, and is often repeated every 2-3 years, with new references required each time. For TM providers who may be required to care for patients in many small rural hospitals or clinics because the rural populations are small and scattered across one or more states the credentialing process is onerous and time wasting. A national credentialing process would improve efficiencies. Some insurance companies already use one national credentialing agency to solve this problem. Delayed credentialing often leads physicians to take jobs in urban areas because they need to work and pay their bills.

   2. **Licensing physicians** by individual State licensing Boards is slow and inefficient. Physicians in the USA are more mobile than ever before. They move State to State due to changing their own jobs or they relocate because of a spouse/partner. TM physicians are hit hard by having to go through licensing in each individual State which can take 3 to 9 months. Most TM providers have to be licensed in multiple states and have to re-license every two years with new letters of reference, and proof of continuing medical education activities which are different for every state. The costs are significant and are a barrier to physicians working in TM. Australia established a National Registration and Accreditation physician system in 2010 to solve this problem.
   In the United States, The Federation of State Medical Boards (FSMB) established the Federation Credentialing Verification (FCVS) system to streamline physician licensing. Thirteen States already require FCVS but five State's won't accept FCVS physician packets. A more comprehensive national licensing system would improve access to healthcare, encourage more physicians to care for rural patients via TM and would lower health system costs. In 2015 the FSMB launched the Interstate Medical License "Compact" which seeks to facilitate a streamlined system for licensing physicians. This has potential to save time but unfortunately physicians still have to go through all the individual State licensing process and pay all the individual State licensing fees which for physicians who work across State lines (TM or in person) is very time consuming and expensive.

   In closing, I thank the committee for its attention to this significant issue and for allowing me to present my thoughts on the potential impact of Telemedicine on economic vitality of Rural America.

Testimony of Michael P. Adcock
Executive Director, Center for Telehealth
University of Mississippi Medical Center

House Small Business Committee
Subcommittee on Agriculture, Energy, and Trade
Subcommittee on Health and Technology
July 20, 2017

Chairman Blum, Chairman Radewagen, Ranking Member Schneider, Ranking Member Espaillat, and Members of the Small Business Committee, thank you for the opportunity to appear before the subcommittees today. I am Michael Adcock, Executive Director for the Center for Telehealth at the University of Mississippi Medical Center (UMMC) in Jackson, Mississippi. I am honored to talk to you this morning about telehealth and the ways its power can be harnessed to address the healthcare needs of America's small businesses.

Mississippi has significant healthcare challenges, leading the nation in heart disease, obesity, cardiovascular disease and diabetes. These and other chronic conditions require consistent, quality care—a task that is made harder by the rural nature of our state. In order to improve access to care and give Mississippians a better quality of life, it is clear we need something more than traditional, clinic and hospital-based services.

Telehealth has been a part of the healthcare landscape in Mississippi for over 13 years, beginning with an aggressive program to address mortality in rural emergency departments. In 2003, three rural sites were chosen to participate in a program that would allow UMMC board certified emergency medicine physicians to interact with and care for patients in small, rural emergency rooms via a live, two way, audio-video connection. The TelEmergency program has grown to serve more than 20 hospitals and continues to produce outcomes on par with that of our Level 1 trauma center. This program has had a significant impact, not only in bringing quality care to the residents of the community, but in supporting the viability of the community hospitals themselves. As a result of TelEmergency, rural hospitals are able to identify and recruit healthcare professionals who live in the community and desire to work locally. The program helps communities retain healthcare revenue that was lost as a result of patients being transferred out for care. In some cases, Telemergency prevented hospital closures that would been detrimental to these underserved communities. The success of this program and noteworthy outcomes led to the development of additional healthcare models using technology to address needs statewide.

Today, the UMMC Center for Telehealth delivers more than 30 medical specialties in over 200 sites across the state including rural clinics, schools, prisons and corporations. It is important to note that a very small portion of these sites are actual UMMC sites. As every community has different needs, we partner with local providers to address their specific needs. UMMC is committed to supporting the community providers through collaborative models that promote efficient use of vulnerable resources. The depth and breadth of our statewide network allows us to deliver world-class care in 68 of our state's 82 counties and provides access for patients who might otherwise go untreated. Over the last decade, we have conducted over 500,000 patient encounters through telehealth. Maximizing our utilization of healthcare resources through the use of technology is the only way we can reach all of the Mississippians who need lifesaving health care.

Small businesses account for 99.9% of all firms in the United States and 96.2% of all Mississippi businesses. The one year survival rate for small businesses averages 78.5%. Approximately half of these establishments survive five years. In Mississippi, the small business exit rate is higher than the startup rate. Small businesses often site access to affordable healthcare as their number one concern. According to the Gallup-Healthways Well-Being Index, annual costs for local productivity for employees having chronic conditions totaled $84 billion. Multiple publications site that unschedule absenteeism costs roughly $3,600 per year for each hourly worker and $2,650 for each salaried employee. These factors lead to over $250 billion in lost economic output per year in the United States.[1]

Decreasing absenteeism, increasing productivity and improving access to high quality care were the drivers behind the creation of the eCorporate and eSchool Health programs at UMMC. The eCorporate service allows employees to access high quality care from their workplace through secure audio/visual connections. This program is employee initiated and avoids travel to seek medical care, promotes appropriate use of healthcare resources and is a lower cost alternative to the higher cost healthcare settings.

UMMC's eCorporate program is unique in that it is not designed to be a standalone means for primary care, but as an additional avenue for employees to access safe healthcare in an affordable and convenient manner. In many cases, this program has helped identify healthcare needs that, if gone untreated, would have resulted in increased healthcare burden and loss of productivity. For this reason, several corporations have chosen to pay for this service for their employees and allow paid time during the workday to use the service, further reducing barriers to health care. Healthcare is a collaborative effort, and this program is no different. Should an employee have a need outside the scope of telehealth, UMMC assists in securing appropriate follow up with local providers. The goal is to refer locally and support the local community when possible. The eCorporate program currently covers more than 4,000 employees and dependents in businesses across Mississippi We have customers with as few as 15 employees. When you add our program for State Employees (UMMC 2 You), we cover over 185,000 lives across our state.

Our corporate offerings are not only aimed at patient initiated services. We currently offer wellness services and diabetes prevention/management services for corporations across Mississippi. We are working with some businesses to augment their current wellness services by helping to risk stratify their employees' annual

---

[1] U.S. Small Business Administration, Office of Advocacy

lab work and biometric measurements. This leads to proactive visits with our providers to discuss risk factors and wellness. The goal is to educate these employees on healthy living and how they can address their risk factors to live a healthier life.

Similarly, the eSchool Health program provides the school nurse with additional provider support needed to reduce absenteeism and improve student performance. With very few local primary care providers, nurses and parents have difficulty ensuring that students will have access to basic, and sometimes vital health services. With eSchool Health, school districts partner with UMMC to provide a more comprehensive health care offering that can assist with health care related needs such as asthma action plans and medication refills. Our eCorporate and eSchool Health programs are examples of working with community leaders to create an environment that is attractive to business by supporting efforts to produce healthy families.

Another program that has been very impactful for patients is remote patient monitoring (RPM), which supports patients as they manage chronic disease in their homes. RPM is designed to educate, engage and empower patients so that they can learn to take care of themselves. Our initial pilot with diabetics in the Mississippi Delta was a public/private partnership between critical access hospital North Sunflower Medical Center, telecommunications provider C Spire, technology partner Care Innovations, the Mississippi Division of Medicaid, Office of the Governor of Mississippi and UMMC. The purpose of the pilot was to test the effectiveness of remote patient monitoring using technology in a rural, underserved area. Specifically, the desired outcome was to reduce Hemoglobin A1C by 1% in uncontrolled diabetics. The participants in this study received their healthcare in the local and rural health clinic. UMMC supported these providers by delivering diabetic education, monitoring biometrics and serving as a liaison between the patient and their provider as they learn to manage their condition. The preliminary results through six months of the study showed: a marked decrease in blood glucose, early recognition of diabetes-related eye disease, reduced travel to see specialists and no diabetes-related hospitalizations or emergency room visits among our patients. This pilot demonstrated a savings of over $300,000 in the first 100 patients over six months. The Mississippi Division of Medicaid extrapolated this data to show potential savings of over $180 million per year if 20 percent of the diabetics on Mississippi Medicaid participated in this program.

Given the success of the diabetes pilot, UMMC Center for Telehealth has expanded remote patient monitoring to other disease states, including adult and pediatric diabetes, congestive health failure, hypertension, bone marrow transplant and kidney transplant. Working closely with a patient's primary care provider, we continue to grow this program both in terms of volume and number of diseases that can be managed. Most importantly, this program is giving patients the knowledge and tools they need to improve their health and manage their chronic disease. Businesses that are a part of our eCorporate program are also given the option to provide this service to their high risk employees with chronic disease.

The employers see this as a way to offer their employees additional support and to reduce costs incurred for after hour clinic visits and emergency room visits for non-emergent conditions. Many small businesses are self-insured, so a program of this type provides quality care at an affordable rate is attractive and beneficial.

Health care is a major economic driver across the United States, with the sector growing at over 20% annually. In Mississippi, hospitals boast over 60,000 full time employees and create an additional 34,000 outside of their facilities. Every new physician crates approximately 21 jobs and more than $2,000,000 in revenue for a community [2]. Critical Access Hospitals (CAH) are located in small, rural communities and are an important part of the health system. They are responsible on average for 170 jobs with $7.1 million in wages salaries and benefits. For every job in a hospital, an additional .34 jobs are created in other businesses in the local economy. This means that the average CAH is responsible for an additional 43 jobs outside of the hospital and $1.8 million of taxable retail sales [3].

Our telehealth program directly supports the financial viability of the health care system, especially primary care providers' offices, small rural hospitals and rural health clinics. Supporting these small businesses also supports the overall financial viability of the community. Collaboration between the Center for Telehealth and providers throughout the state allow for the delivery of high quality specialty care in locations that are convenient for patients. These collaborations deliver multiple benefits: access to specialty care close to home, continuity of care and originating site fees to the local providers. These services do not cost the patients any more than traditional visits, but save them a tremendous amount of time and money on travel. For the clinics, we are able to bring a more comprehensive healthcare offering to their community. Keeping services in communities not only supports the local providers, but keeps much needed employment and revenue in rural communities.

Businesses in Mississippi that have utilized our telehealth and remote patient monitoring programs have demonstrated success by improving access to care, decreasing cost of care and improving quality of care for their employees. Healthy employees mean decreased absenteeism, increase productivity and a greater chance for small businesses to remain viable.

Thank you for your time and attention to this very important matter.

---

[2] Critical Care, The Economic Impact of Hospitals on Mississippi's Economy, 2012
[3] **Economic Impact of a Critical Access Hospital on a Rural Community** Gerald A. Doeksen, Cheryl F. St. Clair, and Fred C. Eilrich, National Center for Rural Health Works

Written Testimony

By

David F. Schmitz, MD

National Rural Health Association, President

On behalf of the National Rural Health Association

For the

United States House

Committee on Small Business

Subcommittee on Health and Technology

July 20, 2017

Good morning, Mr. Chairman, Ranking Member Velázquez, and members of the Subcommittee. Thank you for inviting me here to testify. I am Dr. David Schmitz, a family physician who has practiced and taught in rural America for 20 years. I am here today representing the National Rural Health Association where I currently serve as president. I am grateful for this opportunity to discuss rural health care and its impact on rural America and local economies.

NRHA's mission is to improve the health and wellbeing of all rural Americans and as such, we recognize the important role that health care serves in the economic development of rural communities across the country. The economic needs of rural America are vastly different than those faced by counterparts in other geographic and population settings. So too are the health care challenges, and opportunities, for rural health care providers.

Today I will discuss some of the unique challenges to health care in rural America. I will discuss how rural America has also faced unique economic challenges, and how strong rural health care providers can rise to those challenges by providing direct jobs, stimulating indirect jobs, supporting the growth of employers in other industries, and bolstering entire rural communities.

I am here today to talk about the investments that we need to make to ensure that rural health care thrives and, in return, rural economies thrive and sustain our communities. NRHA believes that improving access to care by investing in rural health care—from workforce to technology infrastructure—is a means to bolster the local economy. This must be a priority for both the Administration and Congress.

Barriers and Challenges of Rural Health Care

For the 62 million Americans living in rural and remote communities, access to quality, affordable health care is a major concern. Rural Americans on average are older, sicker and poorer than their urban counterparts. They are also more likely to suffer from chronic diseases that require monitoring and follow-up care.

Local care is necessary to ensure patient ability to adhere to treatment plans, to help reduce the overall cost of care, and to improve patient outcomes and their quality of life. Whether following delivery of a baby or a significant loss of function due to stroke, locally integrated care for rural people and their own support system is not only the right care, it's better care. Rural communities are resourceful and continuity of care is primary to good outcomes such as avoidance of hospital re-admission. Investing dollars locally can save many more otherwise wasted dollars lost to inefficiencies, anonymity and the gaps that occur in the miles between.

There is no doubt that rural health care delivery is challenging. Workforce shortages, older and poorer patient populations, geographic barriers, low patient volumes and high rates of publicly insured Medicare and Medicaid recipients, uninsured and underinsured populations are just a few of the barriers.[1]

Unfortunately, a growing number of rural Americans are living in areas with limited health care options. Indeed, 81 rural hospitals have closed since 2010, leaving many rural Americans without timely access to emergency care. The two most recent of these, closing on June 30th of this year, are in Florida and Texas. The majority rural closures are in states that did not expand Medicaid, and with reductions in the Disproportion Share (DSH) payments that helped hospitals cover bad debts incurred by serving high rates of uninsured people, these hospitals could not survive.[2,3,4,5,6] There are 673 additional rural hospitals that are on the brink of closure.

The health disparities between rural populations and their urban counterparts are pronounced. This can be particularly true among the growing minority populations in rural America. A recent study in the *Journal of Rural Health* underscored the alarming extent of these challenges.

Using data from the National Center for Health Statistics, and adjusting for age, the researchers found that rural whites have 102 more deaths per 100,000 members of the population than their urban counterparts. Rural blacks have 115 more deaths per 100,000 than their urban counterparts. The number of excess rural deaths from 1986 to 2012 was 694,000 for whites and 53,000 for blacks.[7]

Economic Impact of Rural Providers

Rural health care providers are not only critically important for the health of rural Americans, the providers are critically important for the economic health of rural communities.

Much of rural America was left behind in the economic recovery. According to the United States Department of Agriculture (USDA), rural counties were losing 200,000 jobs per year and the rural unemployment rate stood at nearly 10 percent during the Great Recession. Since then, economic recovery hasn't returned to rural America. In fact, 95% of the jobs that have returned after the Great Recession have been to urban, not rural areas.

While many industries in rural America have been shrinking, for a wide variety of reasons, health care is an industry with the potential to reverse declining employment. As factory and farming jobs decline, the local rural hospital often becomes the hub of the local business community—not only offering critical life-saving services, but representing as much as 20 percent of the rural economy.

Simply put, hospitals provide a large number of jobs. The economic wellbeing of rural American towns depends on a healthy rural economy, which is anchored by the local rural hospital and local provider. The average Critical Access Hospital (CAH) creates 195 jobs and generates $8.4 million in payroll annually. Rural hospitals are often the largest or second-largest employer in a rural co9mmunity (along with the school system). In addition, even a single rural primary care physician can generate 23 jobs and more than $1 million in annual wages, salaries and benefits.[8]

Because hospitals provide so many jobs, it follows that their closure has a devastating effect on employment. If Congress allows the 673 additional vulnerable rural hospitals to shut their doors, 99,000 direct health care jobs and another 137,000 community jobs will vanish.

A critical component of maintaining economic stability in rural communities is ensuring that rural hospitals and other health care providers are able to remain in their communities. Protecting rural hospitals from closure is an immediate step that can be taken to prevent significant job loss in rural communities.

Workforce challenges also exist in rural America. The rural health landscape with its uneven distribution and shortage of health care professionals is faced with significant problems in recruiting and retaining a trained health care workforce. This is compounded by the disparity in federal reimbursement for rural providers, which if addressed, would not only improve the recruitment and retention of rural physicians, but would also stabilize the rural economy.

Providers are more likely to practice in a rural setting if they have a rural background, participate in a rural training program (RTT Technical Assistance Program) and have a desire to serve rural community needs. The RTT Technical Assistance Program [9] identified that residents training in rural training track residency programs were about twice as likely to practice in rural areas following graduation than family medicine graduates overall.[10] Likewise, an emphasis on inter-professional education, rural medical school tracks, admission of rural and minority students to health professions education are all part of the workforce solution. Training doctors and other health professionals close to home makes it more likely they will call that place home. Investments in rural distributed medical education are supported by such programs as Area Health Education Centers (AHES),[11] and supported by organizations such as the RTT Collaborative, a not-for-profit sustainable result of the RTT Technical Assistance Program.

To train and educate physicians who will practice in rural, the presence of hospitals and clinics in these rural communities must be present to become part of the "rural medical education campus." Distributed medical education campuses across rural states and rural America then become the platform for workforce initiatives that work, develop infrastructure to support quality healthcare delivery and produce economic value. Graduate medical education regulatory reform that allows for common sense investment specifically allowing for education of physicians in rural hospitals is one example of how to address rural economic development and workforce shortages in one action, while improving quality and delivering cost-saving healthcare.

The Local Scale: How a Healthy Population Means a Healthy Economy

The benefits of strong rural health care providers spread far beyond the number of people directly employed in a hospital.

Consider the case of Beatrice, Nebraska, a rural town in Gage County, Nebraska. The town has a burgeoning economy largely thanks to the Beatrice Hospital, a CAH with 25 beds, and its related health services. Beatrice is an example of how related health care services flourish when a strong local hospital is nearby. In Beatrice, home health services and assisted living homes have sprung up around the hospital to fulfill the necessary care for the town's elderly (the town's average age is six years higher than the state of Nebraska's average age).

Beatrice Hospital shows how significant the direct and indirect effects of a good hospital are for rural communities. Beatrice Hospital is the town's largest employer with 512 workers. Its payroll is nearly $28 million, and the average starting salary for a nurse is $40,000.

The wages provided by the hospital's good jobs circulate throughout the local economy, stimulating small businesses, the local real estate market and more in a virtuous circle for the community. That's why across the country, small rural towns like Beatrice, "have emerged as oases of economic stability across the nation's heartland."[12]

Rural hospitals provide other types of indirect stimulus as well. A hospital's construction and maintenance requires non-hospital-affiliated labor and external contractors to complete. In order to build and maintain a hospital, and receive these benefits, investment in local resources and labor are necessary.

One way to quantify the total impact of the indirect economic benefits of rural hospitals is using employment and labor multipliers. These multipliers are used to measure job and revenue creation upon the entrance of a hospital into a specific market.

If a hospital has an employment or labor multiplier greater than one, it has a positive indirect economic impact. For instance, an employment multiplier of 1.35 would mean that a 100-employee hospital also creates 35 new, non-health-related jobs for local economy. The typical CAH has an employment multiplier of 1.38.

An alternate approach is to look at the multiplier on wages and salaries. For instance, the average wages multiplier for rural hospitals is estimated at 1.24. That means that a rural hospital with $10 million in wages, indirectly generates an additional $2.4 million in local salaries and incomes outside the hospital.

Consider what these multipliers mean for a hospital like the one in Beatrice. The 512-direct jobs generate 179-indirect jobs across the community. The $28 million in direct wages generates $6.7 million in additional wages throughout the community.

And, in Apalachicola, Florida, the George E. Weems Memorial Hospital is a 25-bed Critical Access Hospital that not only provides dynamic health care services to Franklin County and the surrounding area, but it also has an employment multiplier of 1.40. The $1.8 million in local retail sales attributed to hospital generates significant sales tax collection.

The multipliers for other types of rural hospitals are similar. The economics are clear that rural hospitals are powerful engines for boosting job creation and increasing earnings across a rural community.

Locating and Expanding Businesses in Rural

The quality of a community's local health care system is a key factor for firms that are considering where to relocate or expand. Access to quality health care is the number two priority for firms who are making decisions on relocation and expansion. The only thing more important to firms is having access to a skilled workforce.

Without local access to care, the rural economy struggles to grow and thrive. When a community loses access to local health care, it affects the ability of all businesses in the community to go about their business and grow. It is difficult for companies to attract workers with young or expanding families when care for a sick child is not available locally, or if the family must travel hours for prenatal and maternity care.

Knowing you have an emergency room nearby to treat your employees is essential for many businesses, especially within sectors such as farming or energy. The difficult work behind producing our food and energy supply is vital to our nation's economy. This work, which must often be performed in rural and remote areas, has intrinsic risks and dangers. Workers in these vital sectors of the American economy need and deserve access to quality and affordable health care.

Technology such as telemedicine for consultation services have supported rural delivery of care but depend on the adequate development of broadband internet into rural and remote areas. Networks developed for education and building technology-based "virtual communities" can share of best practices and an example such as with Project ECHO will continue to bring more support to rural hospitals and clinics. Still, hands-on care is needed when an unexpected car accident or early delivery of a newborn baby occurs in rural America, no matter if you are a local resident or visiting. Each one of us who spend time and dollars in rural communities will appreciate quality, local care in those moments.

Access to health care is related to the sustainability of small businesses, another hallmark of healthy economies. A rural community simply cannot attract entrepreneurial investment and talent—or entice native talent to remain—without appropriate health services. Small business leaders contribute jobs and more circulating dollars, infusing rural economies with increased assets.

Supporting the Whole Community

The town of Jefferson, Illinois is a testament to the role of a hospital in economic growth. Rand Fisher, president of the Iowa Area Development Group, asserts, "To be successful in business development today, we believe you also have to be very focused on community development."

Fisher is referring to the multi-pronged approach that development-minded communities must take. They must focus on industrial retention, recruitment and entrepreneurship, and community betterment that provides better access to education and health care. A rural hospital is one agent that fulfills all these roles.

Jefferson is "drawing new residents and keeping existing ones through strong business and community development programs," not least of which is its recent hospital renovation. A technological investment introduced state-of-the-art equipment and improved facilities that are better able to serve patients.[13]

Rural hospitals provide cost-effective primary care. It is 2.5 percent less expensive to provide identical Medicare services in a rural setting than in an urban or suburban setting. This focus on primary care, as opposed to specialty care, saves Medicare $1.5 billion per year. Quality performance measurements in rural areas are on par with if not superior to urban facilities. Additionally, CAHs represent nearly 30 percent of acute care hospitals but receive less than 5 percent of total Medicare payments.

When a rural hospital closes or a physician leaves, businesses, families, and retirees are forced to leave. Often, rural physicians are hospital-based. When the hospitals close, the physicians leave, soon followed by nurses, pharmacists and other providers. Medical deserts are forming across rural America. Hundreds of rural jobs are lost, home values drop, and those who can't sell their home are stuck in a dying town that can no longer meet their basic needs. A study shows that "the closure of a rural county's sole hospital decreases the economic well-being of the community and likely places the local economy in a downward cycle that may be very difficult to recover from."[14]

All of these examples show why a strong rural health care system is vital to our states' economies. The rural health care system provides a large number of direct jobs, a large number of indirect jobs, and provides key support for every business in a local community. We have seen the devastating impact that the Great Recession has had on rural communities across the country. Health care is one industry capable of playing a critical role supporting the local economy, and protecting rural communities from further economic damage. If roads and Internet access are the blood vessels and nerves, then health care is the backbone to investing in rural America.

Recommendations

When rural hospitals and providers thrive, so do the physical and fiscal health of the community. The following are NRHA's recommendations:

    1. **H.R. 2957, the Save Rural Hospitals Act.** Passage of this important bill will provide immediate relief to rural hospitals by stopping the onslaught of reimbursement cuts that have hit rural hospitals. Without increasing reimbursement rates, it will stabilize payments and stop rural hospital closures. It will also create a new health care delivery model that

is flexible for the many varied needs in rural communities. Hospitals are essential to rural communities, not just for access to emergency care but for the high-quality jobs supported by the hospital. If the hospital closes, these rural communities will likely face higher poverty rates.

2. **Education:** Continue to fund health workforce programs to not simply recruit individuals to rural areas but to reward those individuals that stay for extended periods of time in these communities. Regulatory reforms related to rural graduate medical education can have a near-term positive effect on workforce and rural economic growth.

3. **Rural Health Networks:** Expand funding for the creation of rural health networks with the intention of identifying innovative strategies to expand services to all residents through access to quality care at a local integrated level, lower costs and a better patient experience.

4. **Research:** The federal government should support research that explores the linkages between a strong healthcare system and sustainable local economies in rural communities.

5. **Technology Infrastructure:** Provide access to capital through grants and loans for facilities to adopt new technology for Electronic Medical Records (EMRs) and to meet all stages of meaningful use. In addition, provide educational programs to train doctors, nurses and other staff not just how to use the technology but how to interpret the data and how to make recommendations for quality improvement. Broadband access in rural America teamed with health professions education access and ongoing support of practice reduces professional isolation, sustains workforce and improves quality.

6. **Telehealth:** Rural providers and other agencies are seeking to implement new medical technologies to enhance quality and delivery of medical care. Telehealth is an example of one of the most important technologies for rural providers. In 2013, over 40,000 rural beneficiaries received at least one telemedicine visit, and this number is expected to continue to grow. If rural providers are to move toward an online future, they must invest in necessary technological infrastructure and systems. Government grants and private investment in technological advancements can increase the flow of new dollars into rural economies, empowering local resources to further health infrastructure.

The National Rural Health Association appreciates the opportunity to provide our testimony and recommendations to the subcommittee. An investment in the rural health delivery system is important to maintaining access to high quality care in rural communities and to a healthy, vibrant economy. We greatly appreciate the support of the subcommittee and look forward to working with members of the subcommittee to continue making these important investments for rural America.

Citations

1. Scotti, S. (2017). Tracking rural hospital closures. *NCSL Legisbrief, 25*(21), 1-2.
2. Blavin, F. (2016). Association Between the 2014 Medicaid Expansion and US Hospital Finances. *JAMA, 316*(14), 1475-1483. doi:10.1001/jama.2016.14765
3. Camilleri, S. (2017). The ACA Medicaid Expansion, Disproportionate Share Hospitals, and Uncompensated Care. *Health Serv Res*. doi:10.1111/1475-6773.12702
4. Dranove, D., Gartwaite, C., & Ody, C. (2017). The Impact of the ACA's Medicaid Expansion on Hospitals' Uncompensated Care Burden and the Potential Effects of Repeal. *Issue Brief (Commonw Fund), 12*, 1-9.
5. Kaufman, B. G., Reiter, K. L., Pink, G. H., & Holmes, G. M. (2016). Medicaid Expansion Affects Rural And Urban Hospitals Differently. *Health Aff (Millwood), 35*(9), 1665-1672. doi:10.1377/hlthaff.2016.0357
6. Wishner J, Solleveld P, Rudowitz R, Paradise J, & Antonisse L. (2016). *A Look at Rural Hospital Closures and Implications for Access to Care: Three Case Studies*. Retrieved from http://files.kff.org/attachment/issue-brief-a-look-at-rural-hospital-closures-and-implications-for-access-to-care
7. James, W. and Cossman, J. S. (2017), Long-Term Trends in Black and White Mortality in the Rural United States: Evidence of a Race-Specific Rural Mortality Penalty. The Journal of Rural Health, 33: 21–31.
8. Eilrich, F. C., Doeksen, G. A., & St. Clair, C. F. (2013). *The Economic Impact of a Rural Primary Care Physician*(Rep.). Stillwater, OK: National Center for Rural Health Works.
9. Rural Health Research Gateway. (n.d.). Retrieved July 17, 2017, from https://www.ruralhealthresearch.org/projects/100002349
10. Patterson DG, Schmitz D, Longenecker R, Andrilla CHA. Family medicine Rural Training Track residencies: 2008-2015 graduate outcomes. Seattle, WA: WWAMI Rural Health Research Center, University of Washington. Feb 2016
11. About: Health Careers Promotion and Preparation. (n.d.). Retrieved July 17, 2017, from http://www.nationalahec.org/programs/HealthCareersRecruitmentandPreparation.html
12. Searcy, D. (2015, April 29). Hospitals Provide a Pulse in Struggling Rural Towns. *The New York Times*. Retrieved July 11, 2017, from https://www.nytimes.com/2015/04/30/business/economy/hospitals-provide-a-pulse-in-struggling-rural-towns.html
13. *Reviving Mainstreet: How Rural Iowa Stays Relevant*(Rep.). (2017). Des Moines, IA: Iowa Association of Businesses and Industry.
14. Holmes, G. M., Slifkin, R. T., Randolph, R. K., & Poley, S. (2006). The Effect of Rural Hospital Closures on Community Economic Health. *Health Services Research, 41*(2), 467–485. http://doi.org/10.1111/j.1475-6773.2005.00497.x

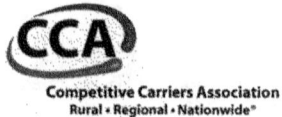

Competitive Carriers Association
Rural • Regional • Nationwide®

July 20, 2017

The Honorable Rod Blum
Chairman
Subcommittee on Agriculture,
 Energy, and Trade
House Small Business Committee
2361 Rayburn House Office Building
Washington, D.C. 20515

The Honorable Brad Schneider
Ranking Member
Subcommittee on Agriculture
 Energy, and Trade
House Small Business Committee
2069 Rayburn House Office Building
Washington, D.C. 20515

The Honorable Aumua Amata Radewagen
Chairwoman
Subcommittee on Health and Technology
House Small Business Committee
2361 Rayburn House Office Building
Washington, D.C. 20515

The Honorable Al Lawson
Ranking Member
Subcommittee on Health and Technology
House Small Business Committee
2069 Rayburn House Office Building
Washington, D.C. 20515

Dear Chairman Blum, Ranking Member Schneider, Chairwoman Radewagen and Ranking Member Lawson:

Competitive Carriers Association (CCA)[1] respectfully submits this letter for the record regarding the joint hearing on "21st Century Medicine: How Telehealth Can Help Rural Communities" by the Subcommittees on Agriculture, Energy, and Trade and Health and Technology. Today's important hearing builds upon last month's hearing on "Improving Broadband Deployment: Solutions for Rural America" and explores one of many key services only available through robust mobile broadband service. As you and your colleagues consider the role of technology in modern health care, we ask that Congress support policies that foster ubiquitous mobile broadband deployment, especially in rural America where patients stand to benefit immensely from new telehealth innovations.

Telemedicine is revolutionizing patient care and eliminating the distance between patients and providers. What's more, remote patient monitoring, provided over competitive carrier networks, is saving costs and reducing hospital visits. Competitive carriers serve some of the most rural parts of the country, and many CCA members help bring telehealth services to their communities. For example, several CCA members provide remote access to doctors through programs like iSelectMD, where patients call a toll-free number or visit the mobile health portal to instantaneously connect with a doctor, increasing access and reducing costs and copays. As another example, ChatMobility launched

---

[1] CCA is the nation's leading association for competitive wireless providers and stakeholders across the United States. CCA's membership includes nearly 100 competitive wireless providers ranging from small, rural carriers serving fewer than 5,000 customers to regional and national providers serving millions of customers. CCA also represents close to 200 associate members, including vendors and suppliers that provide products and services throughout the mobile communications ecosystem. The vast majority of CCA's members are small businesses.

the "Heartland Mobile Health" initiative providing a specially-equipped van that offers mobile health services and maintains electronic medical records for communities in remote and rural areas. C Spire also has partnered with the University of Mississippi Medical Center on a diabetes monitoring project that has the potential to save Medicaid over $189 million a year in hospitalization costs. These initiatives bridge the digital health divide in rural America by connecting rural residents with the same medical attention and care as is provided in urban areas.

But these innovations are only possible through robust mobile broadband networks, the technological key that helps make telemedicine possible. As I testified before the Subcommittee on Agriculture, Trade, and Energy last month, CCA members have made progress working to connect all Americans with ubiquitous coverage, but the job is not done. Gaps in service could prove detrimental to patients who rely on mobile broadband networks to maintain their health through telemedicine. Congress can support telemedicine by streamlining challenges to mobile broadband infrastructure deployment. This includes streamlining the siting process and timelines for application review as carriers seek to deploy or upgrade services. Needless red tape, burdens, fees, or open-ended timeframes frustrate efforts to expand mobile broadband. Removing barriers to deployment at federal, state, and local levels by adopting "dig once" and "deemed granted" policies, master applications, and the use of shot clocks also will help competitive carriers meet the needs of unserved and underserved communities. These initiatives are particularly important as carriers work to densify their networks or bring services to high cost areas.

Additionally, competitive carriers need support from the Universal Service Fund (USF) to preserve and expand mobile broadband in areas that are otherwise uneconomical to serve. Congress should support USF policies that use the most accurate and reliable data to determine which areas are eligible for support, based on the consumer experience on the ground. The Federal Communications Commission (FCC) will vote on how to determine areas eligible for support through the Mobility Fund Phase II next month, and Congress should support efforts that use reliable, standardized data to ensure that rural America is not left behind.

Finally, access to spectrum resources is critical to deploying robust mobile broadband networks. The wireless industry is on the brink of a tectonic technological shift. Consumer demand for mobile data is insatiable, and carriers are now looking forward to deploying 5G next-generation technologies. To make this important jump, competitive carriers must have access to low-, mid-, and high-band spectrum to deploy next-generation mobile broadband and, eventually, 5G networks, especially those serving rural and regional areas. Access to spectrum will determine whether competitive carriers, particularly those that primarily serve rural communities, can meet exploding demand for data. Congress should support policies to allocate additional spectrum resources for commercial mobile broadband use for rural America's connectivity, and ensure that carriers that recently won spectrum licenses in the 600 MHz auction can put the spectrum to use as quickly as possible to serve consumers.

Mobile broadband networks are a key economic driver, and are crucial to providing new, innovative telemedicine services and first-class patient care. Policymakers should support mobile broadband deployment to bring the latest technologies and services, including telehealth, to consumers and patients across the United States.

CCA thanks the Subcommittees for their leadership on this important issue, and looks forward to continued engagement. We welcome any questions you may have.

Sincerely,

Tim Donovan
Senior Vice President, Legislative Affairs

CC:

The Honorable Steve Chabot, Chairman, House Small Business Committee
The Honorable Nydia Velázquez, Ranking Member, House Small Business Committee

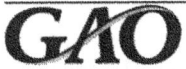

United States Government Accountability Office

Report to Congressional Committees

April 2017

HEALTH CARE

Telehealth and Remote Patient Monitoring Use in Medicare and Selected Federal Programs

GAO-17-365

GAO Highlights

Highlights of GAO-17-365, a report to congressional committees

April 2017

HEALTH CARE

Telehealth and Remote Patient Monitoring Use in Medicare and Selected Federal Programs

Why GAO Did This Study

Telehealth and remote patient monitoring can provide alternatives to health care provided in person at a physician's office, particularly for patients who cannot easily travel long distances for care. Medicare pays for some telehealth services that are subject to statutory and regulatory requirements, such as requiring the patient be present at an originating site like a rural health clinic.

The Medicare Access and CHIP Reauthorization Act of 2015 includes a provision for GAO to study telehealth and remote patient monitoring. Among other reporting objectives, this report reviews (1) the factors that associations identified as affecting the use of telehealth and remote patient monitoring in Medicare and (2) emerging payment and delivery models that could affect the potential use of telehealth and remote patient monitoring in Medicare.

GAO reviewed agency documents and regulations and interviewed agency officials. GAO also selected nine general and medical specialty associations with expertise and interest in telehealth or remote patient monitoring—six provider, two patient, and one payer association—based on a review of relevant documents and literature and through background interviews. GAO interviewed representatives from each of the associations and collected information from the provider and patient associations through a data collection instrument.

GAO provided a draft of this report to HHS. In response, HHS provided technical comments, which were incorporated as appropriate.

View GAO-17-365. For more information, contact Carolyn L. Yocom at (202) 512-7114 or Yocomc@gao.gov.

What GAO Found

Selected associations representing providers and patients most often cited the potential to improve or maintain quality of care as a significant factor that encourages the use of telehealth (providing clinical care remotely by two-way video) and remote patient monitoring (monitoring of patients outside of conventional settings) in Medicare. For example, according to officials from a provider association, telehealth can improve patient outcomes by facilitating follow-up care, while remote patient monitoring is helpful for treating patients with chronic diseases. With regard to factors that create barriers, the selected associations most often cited concerns over payment and coverage restrictions. For example, officials from a provider association noted that Medicare telehealth coverage restrictions limit the geographic and practice settings in which beneficiaries may receive services. While not indicating how significant these factors are to Medicare, officials with a payer association told GAO that they considered these factors—also identified by the provider and patient associations—as either encouraging use or creating barriers to the use of telehealth and remote patient monitoring.

Significance of Improving or Maintaining Quality of Care as a Factor that Encourages the Use of Telehealth and Remote Patient Monitoring in Medicare

	Provider associations						Patient associations	
	A	B	C	D	E	F	G	H
Telehealth	●	◐	●	●	◉	○	●	●
Remote patient monitoring	●	●	●	◉	●	◐	●	●

● A very significant factor that encourages use
◐ A somewhat significant factor that encourages use
○ A factor that encourages use, but not a significant one
✕ Not a factor that encourages use
◉ Did not respond

Source: GAO analysis of a data collection instrument completed by the associations that represent providers and that associations that represent patients. | GAO-17-365

Medicare models, demonstrations, and a new payment program have the potential to expand the use of telehealth and remote patient monitoring. The Centers for Medicare & Medicaid Services, an agency within the Department of Health and Human Services (HHS), supports eight models and demonstrations in which certain Medicare telehealth requirements have been waived, such as requirements for the locations and facility types where beneficiaries can receive telehealth services. For example, the waivers allow beneficiaries to access telehealth in urban areas, or from their homes. Additionally, the use of telehealth and remote patient monitoring in Medicare may change depending on how many clinicians use them as a way to achieve the goals of the new Merit-based Incentive Payment System, which—starting in 2017—will pay clinicians based on quality and resource use, among other things. Under this payment program, clinicians can use telehealth and, in some instances, remote patient monitoring, to help meet the payment program's performance criteria. For example, clinicians could use telehealth to coordinate care or use remote patient monitoring to remotely gather information to determine a patient's proper dose of medication.

United States Government Accountability Office

Contents

Letter		1
	Background	6
	Available Data Show Low Proportions of Beneficiaries Accessing Telehealth; Limited Data Are Available on Remote Patient Monitoring	14
	CMS Uses Routine Claims Review Processes for Telehealth Payments and Is Examining Some Questionable Claims Identified by MedPAC	18
	Selected Associations Report Telehealth and Remote Patient Monitoring May Improve Care for Medicare Beneficiaries, but Cited Coverage and Payment Restrictions as Barriers	21
	CMS Has Various Efforts Underway That Have the Potential to Expand the Use of Telehealth and Remote Patient Monitoring in Medicare	27
	Agency and Third-Party Comments	34
Appendix I	Use of Remote Patient Monitoring by Selected Private Payers	38
Appendix II	Scope and Methodology for Identifying Factors Affecting the Use of Telehealth and Remote Patient Monitoring	41
Appendix III	Medicare Telehealth Services Added and Denied by the Centers for Medicare & Medicaid Services, 2011-2016	45
Appendix IV	Telehealth and Remote Patient Monitoring Reimbursement and Use in Selected State Medicaid Plans	51
Appendix V	Selected Associations' Rating of the Significance of Factors that Affect Telehealth and Remote Patient Monitoring	53
Appendix VI	Medicare Valuation of Remote Patient Monitoring	58

Appendix VII	Examples of Telehealth and Remote Patient Monitoring in Medicare Models and Demonstrations	64
Appendix VIII	GAO Contact and Staff Acknowledgments	66

Tables

Table 1: Summary of Federal Agency Telehealth Services and Originating Sites	13
Table 2: Medicare Telehealth Requirements Waived for Selected Models and Demonstrations	30
Table 3: Telehealth Use by Selected Models and Demonstrations with Waivers of Certain Medicare Requirements	32
Table 4: Potential Factors that Encourage the Use or Are Barriers to the Use of Telehealth or Remote Patient Monitoring in Medicare Used in the Data Collection Instrument	41
Table 5: Telehealth Service Codes Added by the Centers for Medicare & Medicaid Services (CMS), Calendar Years 2011 through 2016	46
Table 6: Telehealth Service Codes Denied by the Centers for Medicare & Medicaid Services (CMS), Calendar Years 2011 through 2016	48
Table 7: Reimbursement and Use of Telehealth and Remote Patient Monitoring in Selected State Medicaid Programs	51
Table 8: Centers for Medicare & Medicaid Services' Innovation Center Categories and Examples of Potential Telehealth and Remote Patient Monitoring Use in Models or Demonstrations	64

Figures

Figure 1: Example of Telehealth Use in Medicare	9
Figure 2: Significance of Certain Factors That Encourage the Use of Telehealth and Remote Patient Monitoring in Medicare, According to Selected Provider and Patient Associations	22
Figure 3: Significance of Certain Barriers to the Use of Telehealth and Remote Patient Monitoring in Medicare, According to Selected Provider and Patient Associations	25

Figure 4: Significance of Factors That Encourage the Use of Telehealth in Medicare, According to Selected Provider and Patient Associations — 54

Figure 5: Significance of Factors That Encourage the Use of Remote Patient Monitoring in Medicare, According to Selected Provider and Patient Associations — 55

Figure 6: Significance of Barriers to the Use of Telehealth in Medicare, According to Selected Provider and Patient Associations — 56

Figure 7: Significance of Barriers to the Use of Remote Patient Monitoring in Medicare, According to Selected Provider and Patient Associations — 57

Abbreviations

ACO	accountable care organization
AMA	American Medical Association
CCO	coordinated care organization
CHIP	state Children's Health Insurance Program
CMS	Centers for Medicare & Medicaid Services
DOD	Department of Defense
HHS	Department of Health and Human Services
MAC	Medicare Administrative Contractor
MedPAC	Medicare Payment Advisory Commission
RUC	American Medical Association/Specialty Society Relative Value Scale Update Committee
VA	Department of Veterans Affairs

This is a work of the U.S. government and is not subject to copyright protection in the United States. The published product may be reproduced and distributed in its entirety without further permission from GAO. However, because this work may contain copyrighted images or other material, permission from the copyright holder may be necessary if you wish to reproduce this material separately.

GAO U.S. GOVERNMENT ACCOUNTABILITY OFFICE
441 G St. N.W.
Washington, DC 20548

April 14, 2017

Congressional Committees

For certain individuals, such as those who live in remote areas or cannot easily travel long distances, access to health care services can be challenging. Telehealth and remote patient monitoring can provide an alternative to health care provided in person at a physician's office.[1] Telehealth can be used to provide clinical care remotely by two-way video for services such as psychotherapy or the evaluation and management of conditions. Remote patient monitoring can be used to monitor patients with chronic conditions, such as those with congestive heart failure, hypertension, diabetes, and chronic obstructive pulmonary disease, and it can also be used as a diagnostic tool, such as for some heart conditions.[2] Although the literature is mixed on the effectiveness of telehealth and remote patient monitoring, a 2016 review of studies by the Agency for Healthcare Research and Quality—an agency within the Department of Health and Human Services (HHS)—found that the most consistent benefit of telehealth and remote patient monitoring occurs when the technology is used for communication and counseling or to remotely monitor chronic conditions such as cardiovascular and respiratory disease, with improvements in outcomes such as mortality, quality of life, and reductions in hospital admissions.[3]

In recent years there have been efforts to increase the use of telehealth and remote patient monitoring in federal health care programs. A federal strategic plan prepared by the Office of the National Coordinator for Health Information Technology within HHS calls for an increased use of

---

[1] For this report, we define telehealth as clinical services that are provided remotely via telecommunications technologies, while remote patient monitoring is a technology to enable monitoring of patients outside of conventional clinical settings, such as in the home. Federal agencies have various definitions for telehealth, and in this report we show how these definitions vary across programs.

[2] See Ashlea Bennett Milburn et al., "The Value of Remote Monitoring Systems for Treatment of Chronic Disease," IIE Transactions on Healthcare Systems Engineering, vol. 4, no. 2 (2014); David P. Kao et al., "Impact of a Telehealth and Care Management Program on All-Cause Mortality and Healthcare Utilization in Patients with Heart Failure," Telemedicine and e-Health, vol. 22, no. 1 (2016).

[3] Department of Health and Human Services, Agency for Healthcare Research and Quality. Telehealth: Mapping the Evidence for Patient Outcomes from Systematic Reviews, Technical Brief Number 26 (Washington, D.C.: June 2016).

telehealth and remote patient monitoring in federal health care programs.[4] Additionally, in the 21st Century Cures Act, enacted in December 2016, Congress expressed an interest in expanding the use of telehealth in Medicare through increasing the types of sites where telehealth can occur.[5]

While Medicare currently uses telehealth primarily in rural areas or regions designated as having a shortage of health professionals, in the future emerging payment and delivery models may change the extent to which telehealth and remote patient monitoring are available and used by Medicare beneficiaries and providers in other areas.[6] The Centers for Medicare & Medicaid Services (CMS), another HHS agency, oversees Medicare payments for telehealth services. According to the Congressional Budget Office, the financial impact of expanding telehealth and remote patient monitoring in Medicare is difficult to predict—it may reduce federal spending if used in place of face-to-face visits, but it may increase federal spending if used in addition to these visits. Beyond the Medicare program, other federal programs, along with some private insurers, also pay for—or provide—some telehealth and remote patient monitoring services.[7]

The Medicare Access and CHIP Reauthorization Act of 2015 included a provision that we study telehealth and remote patient monitoring.[8] In this report we

1. describe the extent to which telehealth and remote patient monitoring are used by Medicare and other federal programs to provide health care services;

2. assess the extent to which CMS oversees telehealth payments in Medicare;

---

[4]See Department of Health and Human Services, Office of the National Coordinator for Health Information Technology, Federal Health IT Strategic Plan 2015-2020.

[5]Pub. L. No. 114-255, § 4012, 130 Stat. 1033 (2016).

[6]For the purposes of this report, we use the term "provider" to refer to physicians and non-physician practitioners, such as physician assistants and nurse practitioners.

[7]Based on a 2016 study, over half of states had some requirement for telehealth coverage in private insurance. Bob Herman, "Virtual Reality: More Insurers Are Embracing Telehealth," Modern Healthcare, vol. 46, no. 8 (2016).

[8]Pub. L. No. 114-10, § 106, 129 Stat. 87, 140-142 (2015).

3. describe the factors associations representing providers and patients rated—and payers cited—as affecting the use of telehealth and remote patient monitoring in Medicare; and
4. describe how emerging payment and delivery models could affect the potential use of telehealth and remote patient monitoring in Medicare.

Our report also describes the use of remote patient monitoring by selected health plans in the private insurance market (see app. I).

To describe the extent to which telehealth and remote patient monitoring are used by Medicare and other federal programs, we reviewed available data, statutes, regulations, and other relevant documentation related to telehealth in Medicare, Medicaid, the Department of Defense (DOD), and the Department of Veterans Affairs (VA).[9] We interviewed agency officials from CMS as well as officials from DOD and VA, because the latter two departments operate federal programs outside of HHS that provide telehealth to their beneficiaries. The work we performed for each program included the following:

- For Medicare, we reviewed a June 2016 Medicare Payment Advisory Commission (MedPAC) report which, among other things, includes an analysis of Medicare telehealth and remote patient monitoring claims for calendar year 2014.[10]

- For Medicaid, we selected a sample of six states—Connecticut, Illinois, Kansas, Mississippi, Montana, and Oregon—to include in our review. We selected states that varied in geography, physical size, percentage of rural population, and other factors related to coverage and reimbursement for health care services. In particular, we considered factors such as the extent to which the state's Medicaid

---

[9]Federal agencies have various definitions for telehealth. A May 2014 study from a federal working group found that across the 26 agencies that participated in the workgroup, there were multiple unique definitions using the terms "telehealth" and "telemedicine." Some agencies' definitions were broad, for example, defining only the overarching clinical interaction, while others included detailed descriptions of the technology involved. The study concluded that with agencies serving different populations and operating under different missions, a uniform definition of telehealth was elusive, though the study also concluded that the definitions overlapped. See Charles R. Doarn et al., "Federal Efforts to Define and Advance Telehealth—A Work in Progress," Telemedicine and e-Health, vol. 20, no. 5 (2014).

[10]We relied on the MedPAC analysis because it analyzed the most recent Medicare data available at the time we conducted our work. See Medicare Payment Advisory Commission, Report to the Congress: Medicare and the Health Care Delivery System, (Washington, D.C.: June 15, 2016), 229-260.

73

program uses different payment systems, whether the state's Medicaid program reimburses for telehealth, the type of locations for providing the services that were allowed, and the type and number of eligible providers. We obtained information about telehealth and remote patient monitoring use for the most recent state fiscal year available from four of the six states that had the information and also interviewed state officials from all six states about the use of telehealth and remote patient monitoring in their state, including any restrictions on and reimbursement for these services.[11] Our findings for these six states cannot be generalized to other states.

- For DOD, we obtained data on the use of telehealth for fiscal year 2015, the most recent fiscal year available, and we interviewed officials about the use of telehealth and remote patient monitoring in DOD's health care program.

- For VA, we reviewed documentation, interviewed officials, and received data on the use of telehealth and remote patient monitoring for fiscal year 2016, the most recent fiscal year available.

To assess the reliability of the program data we used, we interviewed MedPAC officials on how they collected and analyzed Medicare data for their report; we obtained information from DOD and VA on the controls used by the programs to ensure that the data were accurate and complete. Based on these steps we determined that these data were sufficiently reliable for our purposes.

To assess the extent to which CMS oversees telehealth payments in Medicare, we reviewed related agency documentation and interviewed knowledgeable officials about the procedures used to review claims for telehealth services. Additionally, we reviewed MedPAC's report on Medicare telehealth claims for calendar year 2014 and interviewed MedPAC officials to understand the basis for their findings.[12] We

---

[11]Connecticut, Illinois, and Mississippi provided us with information from 2015, and Montana also provided information for 2013 through 2015. The remaining two states—Kansas and Oregon—did not provide us with information about such things as numbers of patients or expenditures for telehealth or remote patient monitoring.

[12]Medicare Payment Advisory Commission, Report to the Congress: Medicare and the Health Care Delivery System.

74

assessed CMS's oversight procedures and the agency's response to MedPAC's findings using federal standards for internal controls.[13]

To describe the factors associations representing providers and patients rated—and payers cited—as affecting the use of telehealth and remote patient monitoring in Medicare, we developed a data collection instrument for three groups of selected associations—six associations that represent providers, two associations that represent patients, and one association that represents payers. The associations representing providers and patients completed our data collection instrument; the payer association did not.[14] To identify these associations, we reviewed relevant documents and literature and conducted interviews to identify relevant general and specialty associations. In the data collection instrument, we requested that the associations rate the significance of potential factors that may encourage the use of telehealth and remote patient monitoring and potential factors that may create barriers to their use. We identified these factors based on background research and initial interviews with two groups with an interest in telehealth. In addition to having the provider and patient associations rate the factors and having the payer association identify them, we also reviewed relevant documentation and interviewed officials from each provider, patient, and payer association using a structured question set to obtain examples, from their perspective, of how these factors can encourage the use of telehealth and remote patient monitoring in Medicare or create barriers to their use. The perspectives we obtained using the data collection instrument, from our document reviews, and during our interviews with association officials provided insights regarding the officials' views on factors that encourage the use of telehealth and remote patient monitoring and factors that are barriers to their use. These perspectives cannot be generalized. See appendix II for more information on our data collection instrument and on our scope and methodology for identifying relevant associations and the factors, including the significance of the factors as rated by the associations.

---

[13]See GAO, Standards for Internal Control in the Federal Government, GAO-14-704G (Washington, D.C.: September 2014); and Standards for Internal Control in the Federal Government, GAO/AIMD-00-21.3.1 (Washington, D.C.: November 1999). Internal control is a process effected by an entity's oversight body, management, and other personnel that provides reasonable assurance that the objectives of an entity will be achieved.

[14]A representative of the payer association we spoke with told us that the association did not have sufficient time to survey its members and could not complete our data collection instrument without doing so. Therefore, we reported separately the payer association's views on factors that encourage the use of, or are barriers to, telehealth and remote patient monitoring.

75

To describe how emerging payment and delivery models could affect the potential use of telehealth and remote patient monitoring in Medicare, we reviewed CMS documents describing and evaluating the models developed by the Center for Medicare & Medicaid Innovation (Innovation Center) to support alternative approaches to health care payment and delivery.[15] We also studied implementation plans created by participants in one of the models, which outlined how the participants planned to use telehealth. We also interviewed knowledgeable agency officials about how telehealth was used in the models and how the models might affect telehealth and remote patient monitoring use in Medicare in the future. Additionally, we examined documents and interviewed CMS officials regarding a new Medicare payment program that allows the use of telehealth—and to some extent remote patient monitoring—to help achieve some of the goals of the payment program.

We conducted this work from March 2016 to April 2017 in accordance with generally accepted government auditing standards. Those standards require that we plan and perform the audit to obtain sufficient, appropriate evidence to provide a reasonable basis for our findings and conclusions based on our audit objectives. We believe that the evidence obtained provides a reasonable basis for our findings and conclusions based on our audit objectives.

Background

The federal government uses telehealth and remote patient monitoring in various health care programs, including the following:

- Medicare, which provides health care coverage for people age 65 or older, certain individuals with disabilities, and individuals with end-stage renal disease;
- Medicaid, a joint federal-state health care financing program for certain low-income and medically needy individuals;
- DOD, which provides services through its regionally structured health care program to active duty personnel and their dependents,

---

[15]In 2010, the Patient Protection and Affordable Care Act created the Innovation Center within CMS to test new approaches to health care delivery and payment—known as models, or in some cases as demonstrations—in order to reduce Medicare, Medicaid, and state Children's Health Insurance Program expenditures while preserving or enhancing quality of care for beneficiaries of the programs. See Pub. L. No. 111-148, §§ 3021, 10306, 124 Stat. 119, 389, 939 (codified at 42 U.S.C. § 1315a).

- medically eligible Reserve and National Guard personnel and their dependents, and retirees and their dependents and survivors; and
- VA, which delivers medical services to veterans primarily through an integrated health care delivery system.

Other federal agencies—within and outside of HHS—also provide grants to promote the use of telehealth.[16]

Medicare Telehealth and Remote Patient Monitoring Requirements

Medicare began paying separately for certain telehealth services after the passage of the Balanced Budget Act of 1997.[17] The statute requires that Medicare, which covers over 50 million beneficiaries, pay for certain telehealth services, including consultations, office visits, and office psychiatry services, that are furnished through a telecommunications system with audio and video equipment permitting two-way, real-time interactive communication between the patient and distant site provider.[18] According to CMS officials, Medicare fee-for-service does not have an explicit definition of remote patient monitoring. Rather, Medicare pays separately for some services that are used to remotely monitor patients, as well as for other remote monitoring bundled with other services. For

---

[16]For example, within HHS, the Health Resources and Services Administration promotes the use of telehealth technologies for health care delivery, education, and health information services through grant programs. It does this to, among other things, improve health care services for medically underserved populations, support the establishment and operation of resource centers that help in implementing telehealth services, and support implementation of telehealth networks to deliver 24-hour emergency department consultation services. Additionally, the U.S. Department of Agriculture administers grants through the Distance Learning and Telemedicine and the Community Connect programs. The Distance Learning and Telemedicine program funds institutions to support advanced telecommunications in health care and education in rural communities and is designed specifically to assist rural communities that would otherwise be without access to learning and medical services over the Internet. The Community Connect program provides financial assistance to state and local governments, federally-recognized tribes, non-profit organizations, and for-profit corporations in rural areas that lack a minimum broadband speed connection.

[17]Pub. L. No. 105-33, § 4206, 111 Stat. 251, 337 (1997).

[18]Separate payment for telehealth services in Medicare fee-for-service are limited to those on CMS's approved list of telehealth services. Plans within Medicare Advantage—the Medicare managed care program—must cover the same telehealth services as those provided through fee-for-service, and the plans must include these costs in their annual bid amounts. However, Medicare Advantage plans can provide additional telehealth benefits not on CMS's approved list to their beneficiaries by using rebate dollars or charging beneficiaries a supplemental premium. Plans must receive CMS approval in order to provide the additional telehealth benefits.

77

example, separate payment may be made for services used to remotely monitor patients' conditions, such as services that use devices to monitor, record, and relay data on a patient's heart activity to a provider for analysis. Additionally, Medicare pays for remote services as bundled parts of other services, such as elements of monthly care management services.

While telehealth visits with providers are conducted from a separate site, Medicare requires that the patient be physically present at a medical facility such as a hospital, rural health clinic, or skilled nursing facility—referred to as the originating site—during the telehealth service.[19] Eligible providers who are furnishing Medicare telehealth services are located at a separate site, known as the distant site, and these providers submit claims in the service area where their distant site is located.[20] The originating site is paid a facility fee—about $25 in calendar year 2017—under the Medicare Physician Fee Schedule for each telehealth service, and the distant site provider is paid the same rate for services delivered via telehealth as they would be paid for the in-person service, as required by statute.[21] (See fig. 1.)

---

[19]By statute, originating sites are limited to those located in rural health professional shortage areas, counties not included in a metropolitan statistical area, and sites participating in a federal telehealth demonstration project (referred to as telemedicine demonstration projects in statute) approved by or receiving funding from the Secretary of Health and Human Services as of December 31, 2000. Eligible originating sites are a physician or provider office, a critical access hospital, a rural health clinic, a federally qualified health center, a hospital, a hospital-based or critical access hospital-based renal dialysis center or satellites, a skilled nursing facility, and a community mental health center.

[20]Eligible telehealth providers in Medicare are physicians, physician assistants, nurse practitioners, clinical nurse specialists, certified registered nurse anesthetists, nurse-midwives, clinical social workers, clinical psychologists, and registered dietitians or nutrition professionals.

[21]Medicare pays for physician and other health professional services based on a list of services and their payment rates, called the Physician Fee Schedule.

Figure 1: Example of Telehealth Use in Medicare

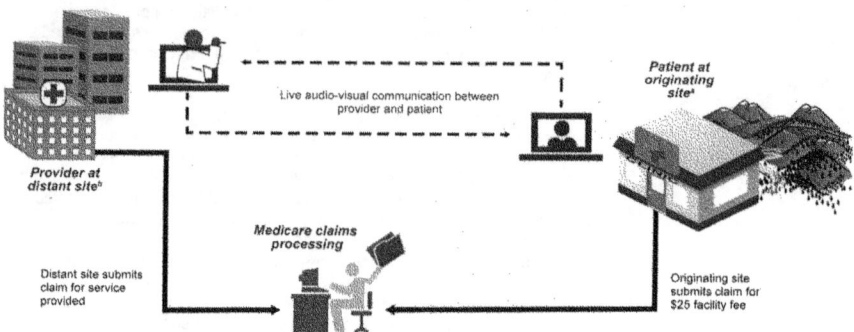

Source: GAO analysis of Medicare statute and regulations. | GAO-17-365

Note: Medicare Administrative Contractors (MAC) process and pay Medicare claims in specific geographic jurisdictions. The MACs review claims and identify and prevent improper payments for Medicare services, including telehealth.

[a] Medicare requires that the patient be physically present at a medical facility—referred to as the originating site—such as a hospital, rural health clinic, or skilled nursing facility during the telehealth service.

[b] Eligible providers who are furnishing Medicare telehealth services are located at a separate site, known as the distant site.

Medicaid, DOD, and VA Telehealth and Remote Patient Monitoring Requirements

CMS does not limit the use of telehealth and remote patient monitoring in Medicaid, which has around 70 million enrollees. Therefore, individual states determine any restrictions and limitations. For example, states have the option to determine

- whether to cover telehealth;
- what types of telehealth to cover;
- how it is provided or covered;
- which types of telehealth providers may be covered or reimbursed, as long as such providers are recognized and qualified according to Medicaid statute and regulation; and

79

- how much to reimburse for telehealth services, as long as such payments do not exceed other requirements.[22]

States are not required to submit a separate state plan amendment to CMS for coverage or reimbursement of telehealth services if they decide to reimburse for telehealth services the same way that they pay for face-to-face services.[23] However, states must submit a separate reimbursement state plan amendment if they want to reimburse for telehealth services or components of telehealth differently than they reimburse for face-to-face services.

DOD, which serves around 9.4 million beneficiaries, allows telehealth through live videoconferencing between the provider and patient at different locations.[24] DOD does not have restrictions on the services that can be provided through its direct care component.[25] Broad types of allowable services include health assessments, treatments, diagnoses, interventions, and consultations. Different categories of providers are allowed to use telehealth and are not required to be individually licensed in the state where the patient—or originating site—is located. These providers include members of the Armed Forces, other DOD uniformed providers, civilian DOD employees, personal services contractors, and National Guard providers who are performing training or duty in response to an actual or potential disaster.[26]

---

[22] For example, there are maximum payment amounts—referred to as the federal upper payment limit—that the federal government will provide in matching funds for reimbursement for services under Medicaid.

[23] Each state has a Medicaid state plan—approved by CMS—that describes, among other things, the services and populations that are covered under the state's Medicaid program.

[24] DOD also uses asynchronous telehealth, called store-and-forward, that involves the capture of diagnostic images, sounds, and data that are interpreted at a later time and at a different location by a qualified diagnostician.

[25] DOD's direct care component provides care in military hospitals and clinics, which are referred to as military treatment facilities. DOD's purchased care, which is care provided through networks of civilian providers, limits services that can be provided via telehealth to clinical consultations, office visits, individual psychotherapy, psychiatric diagnostic interview examination, pharmacologic management, and end-stage renal disease related services when appropriate and medically necessary.

[26] Providers not covered in these categories are required to be licensed in the state where the originating site is located and in the state in which the provider is located when providing such services.

80

DOD allows a range of eligible originating sites for telehealth. In addition to military treatment facilities, eligible originating sites include VA medical centers and clinics; installations, armories, or other non-medical fixed DOD locations; DOD mobile telehealth platforms; civilian sector hospitals and clinics; and contracted provider offices. In February 2016, DOD approved the patient's home as an originating site for telehealth services from providers located in a military treatment facility or other designated facility in DOD's direct care component.[27]

DOD also utilizes remote patient monitoring devices to provide care for eligible beneficiaries for a range of services. These services include the diagnosis and treatment of cardiac conditions, including ambulatory blood pressure monitoring and pacemakers, and continuous glucose monitoring for patients with diabetes. According to DOD officials, the department does not have policies that specifically govern the use of remote patient monitoring devices, but instead DOD leaves the determination of use to clinical practice guidelines or to professional society guidance or recommendations.

VA, which serves about 6.7 million patients, allows the use of telehealth via videoconferencing technologies to enable providers to assess, treat, and provide care to a patient remotely.[28] VA also allows remote patient monitoring using mobile and in-home technologies assigned to veterans

---

[27]In addition to the patient's home, DOD allows telehealth services for any "other patient location" that is deemed appropriate by the treating provider in DOD's direct care component. Among other requirements, the telehealth provider must be privileged at the distant site and must inform the patient's military treatment facility or primary care manager of the care delivered by telehealth. Privileging is the process that health care organizations employ to authorize providers to provide specific services to their patients. In the case of DOD's purchased care, the originating site must be located where the authorized provider normally offers professional medical or psychological services, such as the provider's office.

[28]VA also uses store-and-forward telehealth, which uses devices to capture and store images, sounds, or data that are then forwarded to clinical caregivers for asynchronous review and interpretation.

81

based on individual needs.[29] According to officials, VA does not restrict the use of telehealth or remote patient monitoring by type of service, provider, or location. Telehealth in VA can take place in various originating and distant site locations throughout the country, such as between two VA medical centers; a VA medical center and a community-based outpatient clinic; two community-based outpatient clinics; from the provider's site and the veteran's home, a community living center, or a contract nursing home; and a provider's home and sites such as a VA medical center or community-based outpatient clinic. In recent years, VA has taken steps to increase the use of telehealth. As part of VA's fiscal year 2009 to fiscal year 2013 telehealth transformational initiative, VA recruited over 970 telehealth clinical technicians and purchased equipment for over 900 sites of care.

Table 1 summarizes the use of telehealth and remote patient monitoring in Medicare, Medicaid, DOD, and VA health programs.

---

[29]The remote patient monitoring technologies include VA-provided hub devices placed in the veteran's home, as well as mobile platforms for use with the veteran's own device. The VA-provided hub devices can receive and transmit data via a landline phone, or in homes without a landline via a cellular modem integrated with the device, or by using the veteran's personal computer. Mobile platforms include interactive voice response, which allows veterans to use their own landline or cell phone to receive and transmit responses using voice and keypad entry, and web-enabled technology, allowing veterans to use their own smartphone, computer, or tablet to access a secure VA vendor website for data transmission.

Table 1: Summary of Federal Agency Telehealth Services and Originating Sites

Federal agency		Telehealth services	Originating sites
Centers for Medicare & Medicaid Services (CMS)	Medicare	Medicare pays for the 81 telehealth services on CMS's list of telehealth services as of 2016.	For sites located in a rural health professional shortage area or a county that is not included in a Metropolitan Statistical Area, Medicare pays for telehealth used at the following locations:[a] • physician or provider office, • critical access hospital, • rural health clinic, • federally qualified health center, • hospital, • hospital-based or critical access hospital-based renal dialysis center or satellites, • skilled nursing facility, and • community mental health center.
	Medicaid	Services covered differ depending on the state. According to CMS officials, CMS does not have any statutory or regulatory requirements for telehealth use in Medicaid.	CMS does not limit telehealth use in Medicaid. Restrictions on use vary by state.
Department of Defense (DOD)		DOD does not limit the services allowed for telehealth use within its direct care component.[b]	Outside of military treatment facilities, originating sites are allowed at patient locations that are deemed appropriate by the treating provider in DOD's direct care component, including the patient's home. According to officials, telehealth services are not limited to certain geographic areas, such as rural locations.
Department of Veterans Affairs (VA)		According to officials, VA does not limit the services providers can offer via telehealth.	According to officials, VA does not limit the locations where telehealth services may be offered.

Sources: CMS, DOD, and VA. | GAO-17-365

Note: The term "originating site" refers to the location where the patient is located while receiving a telehealth service.

[a] Medicare also pays for telehealth use for entities that participate in a federal telehealth demonstration project (referred to as telemedicine demonstration projects in statute) approved by or receiving funding from the Secretary of Health and Human Services as of December 31, 2000.

[b] DOD's direct care component provides care in military hospitals and clinics, which are referred to as military treatment facilities. DOD's purchased care, which is care provided through networks of civilian providers, limits services that can be provided via telehealth to clinical consultations, office visits, individual psychotherapy, psychiatric diagnostic interview examination, pharmacologic management, and end-stage renal disease related services when appropriate and medically necessary. Additionally, for purchased care, the originating site must be located where the authorized provider normally offers professional medical or psychological services, such as the provider's office.

Available Data Show Low Proportions of Beneficiaries Accessing Telehealth; Limited Data Are Available on Remote Patient Monitoring

Our review of available data shows that low proportions of beneficiaries received care through telehealth in Medicare, Medicaid, VA, and DOD—from less than 1 percent of beneficiaries in Medicare and DOD to 12 percent in VA—while the types of services available through these technologies varies. Data on use of remote patient monitoring are not aggregated for analysis in Medicare and are not available in selected Medicaid states, and limited data are available for DOD and VA.

Medicare

Telehealth and Remote Patient Monitoring in Medicare

Medicare pays for a limited number of Part B services furnished by a physician or provider to an eligible beneficiary via a telecommunications system. Part B services include physician and outpatient hospital services. For eligible telehealth services, the use of a telecommunications system substitutes for an in-person encounter. According to officials, CMS does not consider remote patient monitoring services as a separate set of services, as it does with telehealth.

Source: CMS. | GAO-17-365

Available calendar year 2014 data show that Medicare providers used telehealth services for a small proportion of beneficiaries and relatively few services. An analysis of Medicare claims data by MedPAC shows that about 68,000 Medicare beneficiaries—0.2 percent of Medicare Part B fee-for-service beneficiaries—accessed services using telehealth.[30] MedPAC also found that 10 states accounted for 42 percent of all Medicare telehealth visits, with South Dakota, followed by Iowa and North Dakota, accounting for the highest use—more than 20 telehealth services were provided per 1,000 fee-for-service beneficiaries.[31] As of 2016, Medicare pays for 81 telehealth services. (See app. III for a list of health care services CMS has added or denied for inclusion on the Medicare list of telehealth services.)

According to MedPAC, beneficiaries accessing telehealth averaged about three telehealth visits per person per year in calendar year 2014, and Medicare spent an average of $182 per beneficiary, for a total of about $14 million. The majority of telehealth visits—62 percent—were for beneficiaries younger than 65 years old.[32] The most common telehealth visits in calendar year 2014 were for evaluation and management services (66 percent), followed by psychiatric visits (19 percent).

---

[30] See Medicare Payment Advisory Commission, Report to the Congress: Medicare and the Health Care Delivery System. Part B services include physician and outpatient hospital services.

[31] The other seven states are—in rank order of use of telehealth per 1,000 beneficiaries—Wyoming, Nebraska, Minnesota, Missouri, Montana, Texas, and Oklahoma.

[32] Medicare provides health care coverage for certain individuals with disabilities and individuals with end-stage renal disease, in addition to people age 65 or older.

MedPAC reported that physicians and nurse practitioners were the most common providers participating in telehealth visits in calendar year 2014 and, of all providers, behavioral health clinicians, including psychiatrists, made up 62 percent of providers at distant sites.[33] According to MedPAC, a small proportion of providers accounted for the majority of telehealth visits in calendar year 2014. Ten percent of distant sites providers accounted for 69 percent of telehealth claims.

According to officials, because CMS does not have a separate category for remote patient monitoring services, as it does with telehealth, and these services may be bundled with other services, CMS has not conducted a separate analysis of remote patient monitoring services. Therefore, the number of Medicare beneficiaries who use this service is unknown. While the number of beneficiaries who use remote patient monitoring is not identified, MedPAC reported information on Medicare spending on remote patient monitoring for selected services. Specifically, MedPAC reported that Medicare spent $119 million on remote cardiac monitoring services for 265,000 beneficiaries in calendar year 2014.[34] MedPAC also reported that in calendar year 2014, Medicare spent $70 million on remote patient monitoring for 639,000 beneficiaries to remotely monitor heart rhythms through implantable cardiac devices, such as pacemakers, and to evaluate the function of these devices.

Medicaid

Telehealth and Remote Patient Monitoring in Medicaid

CMS does not limit the use of telehealth or remote patient monitoring in Medicaid. The use of and any restrictions on telehealth and remote patient monitoring in Medicaid are left up to the states. As a result, states may have varying definitions of telehealth and remote patient monitoring.

Source: CMS. | GAO-17-365

In Medicaid, the use of telehealth and remote patient monitoring varies by state. We interviewed officials from six states and among these officials, the ones from states that were generally more rural than urban said they used telehealth and remote patient monitoring more frequently than officials from more urban states. Officials from four states provided the following information on the use of telehealth and remote patient monitoring in their Medicaid program.

- A Connecticut official said that in the state, which has medical centers in-state and is close to multiple medical centers in other states, Medicaid uses telehealth in a limited capacity by only allowing

---

[33] The distant site is a separate location where the provider furnishing the telehealth service is located.

[34] These services were for mobile cardiac telemetry monitoring of patients to record the patient's electrocardiographic rhythm using external, rather than implantable, devices. The data are sent via phone signal to a surveillance site, and a physician reviews the data and prepares a report.

provider-to-provider consults via secure messaging in federally qualified health centers. According to this official, Connecticut Medicaid data show that the state spent $89,053 on 817 provider-to-provider consults in 2015. The official told us that Connecticut officials needed to be convinced that the use of telehealth would not lead to unnecessary utilization of services in order to expand telehealth reimbursement beyond these consults.

- In Illinois, officials told us that telehealth represented a very small portion of the overall Medicaid budget and was used primarily to provide psychiatric services. According to officials, less than $500,000 of Illinois' $20 billion in Medicaid spending in the state fiscal year 2015 was for telehealth.

- Mississippi began reimbursing for telehealth and remote patient monitoring in January 2015. Mississippi telehealth data show that from January 2015 through June 2015 Medicaid expenditures were about $9,360 for 210 claims for 172 managed care patients and $13,218 for 222 claims for 184 fee-for-service patients. For remote patient monitoring during the same period, Mississippi Medicaid expenditures were about $27,634 for 292 claims for 158 managed care patients and $4,969 for 99 claims for 68 fee-for-service patients.

- Montana officials told us they have used telehealth as a tool to help patients see both in-state and out-of-state specialists remotely, as there is limited access to specialists in the state. According to state officials, Montana's Medicaid spending on telehealth increased from state fiscal years 2013 through 2015. Specifically, according to officials, Montana's Medicaid program spent about $284,675 for 3,218 telehealth distant site claims related to telehealth services provided in state fiscal year 2015, which is an increase from about $132,194 for 1,841 distant site claims in state fiscal year 2013. According to officials, Montana's Medicaid program reimbursed the site where the patient is located about $3,438 for 260 originating site claims in state fiscal year 2015, with psychiatric services accounting for the largest share of the state's Medicaid telehealth expenditures that year.

For more details on telehealth and remote patient monitoring use in Medicaid in the six selected states, see appendix IV.

DOD

Telehealth and Remote Patient Monitoring in DOD

In DOD, synchronous, or "real time," telehealth uses live videoconferencing, with or without additional instrumentation, between provider and patient.

According to DOD officials, the department allows remote monitoring for certain conditions, but does not have policies that specifically govern the use of remote patient monitoring devices, and leaves the determination of use to clinical practice guidelines or professional society guidance or recommendations.

Source: DOD. | GAO-17-365

Fiscal year 2015 data show 25,389 DOD beneficiaries—or about 0.3 percent—received care through telehealth.[35] The most commonly offered telehealth services were behavioral health/psychiatry services, which accounted for approximately 80 percent of all telehealth encounters in fiscal year 2015, followed by dermatology, cardiology, and pediatric services. According to officials, DOD data also show that the top five locations in fiscal year 2015 for the provision of telehealth services were San Antonio, Texas; Fort Shafter, Hawaii; Fort Meade, Maryland; Joint Base Lewis-McChord, Washington; and Landstuhl, Germany. According to DOD officials, of these locations, the surrounding areas of San Antonio, Fort Shafter, and Joint Base Lewis-McChord include zip codes that are considered rural or have an area serviced by a sole community hospital.[36] DOD has also used provider-to-provider e-consultations, which, according to a DOD official, allow providers to give consults to other providers who are deployed or stationed in remote areas, making it easier for providers to consult with one another even when separated by distance. According to officials, DOD also uses remote patient monitoring devices—such as remote pacemaker monitoring and sleep study monitors—to varying degrees across military treatment facilities. DOD officials noted that the agency conducted an Army pilot program using remote patient monitoring for 51 soldiers with known or newly diagnosed Type 1 Diabetes. According to DOD officials, DOD is currently developing additional pilot programs for remote patient monitoring.

VA

Telehealth and Remote Patient Monitoring in VA

Clinical video telehealth uses videoconferencing technologies to allow veterans to connect with their clinical caregivers. We refer to this as telehealth in our report.

Home telehealth monitors veterans using mobile and in-home technologies assigned to veterans based on individual needs. We refer to this as remote patient monitoring in our report.

Source: VA. | GAO-17-365

According to VA officials, VA provided telehealth services to more than 702,000 veterans during fiscal year 2016, or approximately 12 percent of veterans enrolled in VA's health care system. Of these veterans, approximately 45 percent were veterans living in rural areas with limited access to VA health care. Of these 702,000 veterans using telehealth, 150,600 veterans used remote patient monitoring services at least once from October 2015 to September 2016.

VA documents show that VA uses telehealth and remote patient monitoring for a wide range of services. These services include mental health services, such as services for post-traumatic stress disorder;

---

[35]DOD telehealth also includes asynchronous telehealth, called store-and-forward, that involves the capture of diagnostic images, sounds, and data that are interpreted at a later time and at a different location by a qualified diagnostician.

[36]Sole community hospitals provide health care in rural areas or areas where similar hospitals do not exist.

87

primary care; rehabilitation; speech and audiology services; eye care; dermatology services; specialty care; critical care; and care for chronic conditions such as diabetes, chronic heart failure, chronic obstructive pulmonary disease, hypertension, and depression. According to VA officials, providers from over 50 different specialties are using telehealth. VA officials noted that as of May 2016, the most common conditions for veterans using remote patient monitoring were hypertension (almost 19,000 veterans) and diabetes (about 14,000 veterans).

CMS Uses Routine Claims Review Processes for Telehealth Payments and Is Examining Some Questionable Claims Identified by MedPAC

CMS oversees telehealth payments as a part of its general efforts to prevent improper payments in Medicare.[37] CMS relies on Medicare Administrative Contractors (MAC), which process and pay Medicare claims in specific geographic jurisdictions. The MACs review claims to, among other things, identify and prevent improper payments for Medicare services, including telehealth. According to CMS officials, similar to other services, CMS has directed the MACs to only approve and pay claims with a telehealth modifier if the claims meet the statutory and regulatory criteria for covered telehealth services.[38]

According to CMS officials, CMS does not conduct any enhanced oversight or fraud prevention specific to telehealth payments, though officials told us that if there were indications of inappropriate payments or fraud schemes related to telehealth payments, CMS would provide additional oversight for these claims. Telehealth represents a very small percentage of all Medicare claims.[39] CMS requires the MACs to focus

---

[37]An improper payment is any payment that should not have been made or that was made in an incorrect amount (including overpayments and underpayments) under statutory, contractual, administrative, or other legally applicable requirements. This definition includes any payment to an ineligible recipient, any payment for an ineligible good or service, any duplicate payment, any payment for a good or service not received (except where authorized by law), and any payment that does not account for credit for applicable discounts. Improper Payments Elimination and Recovery Act of 2012, Pub. L. No. 112-248, § 3(a)(1), 126 Stat 2390 (codified at 31 U.S.C. § 3321 note).

[38]Distant site providers who furnish telehealth services bill for these services using a GT or GQ code modifier. The GT modifier is used if the telehealth service was provided via interactive audio and video telecommunications systems. The GQ modifier is used if the telehealth service was provided via an asynchronous telecommunications system. The site where the patient is located can also submit a separate originating site claim, which is indicated by the use of code Q3014.

[39]According to MedPAC, in calendar year 2014, Medicare paid 175,000 telehealth claims for a total of about $14 million, which is less than 0.01 percent of the approximately $257 billion in total annual Medicare expenditures on Part B services in fiscal year 2014.

their efforts on areas that pose the greatest financial risk to the Medicare program and where their efforts are likely to produce the best return on investment, which is consistent with federal internal controls.[40]

CMS officials told us that there are no payment incentives for a provider to put a telehealth modifier on a non-approved telehealth service, because the provider could receive payment for that service if it did not include the modifier and the service is payable under Medicare's Physician Fee Schedule. That is, the payment to a distant site provider for a service on the approved telehealth list would be the same amount as the payment for the service if it were furnished in person. Adding a telehealth modifier incorrectly also increases the possibility that claim would be examined, CMS officials said, reducing the incentive to incorrectly add the telehealth modifier. CMS officials also said that for 2017 Medicare is using a new place of service code to describe services furnished via telehealth. According to officials, the code is intended to better identify telehealth services.

However, MedPAC's 2016 report, which examined Medicare telehealth claims, identified potential improper telehealth payments. Specifically, MedPAC reported that among the 175,000 Medicare telehealth claims paid in calendar year 2014, 55 percent, or about 95,000 claims, did not have a corresponding originating site claim.[41] Because there was no originating site claim, it is unclear whether these beneficiaries received telehealth services in a location not permitted under the Medicare statute, such as the home, an originating site located in an urban area, or whether the claims were paid under a demonstration project or model. The Medicare statute requires beneficiaries to receive telehealth services in an originating site located in a rural area, as defined by Medicare for telehealth purposes, unless the site is part of a demonstration project or is participating in a Medicare model where telehealth location requirements are waived.

The absence of a corresponding originating site claim does not definitively indicate that the telehealth claims are improper, though it warrants further review. As a possible explanation for the difference in the number of originating site claims relative to distant site claims, CMS

---

[40]GAO-14-704G, GAO/AIMD-00-21.3.1.

[41]Calendar year 2014 Medicare data were the most complete year of data at the time of MedPAC's review.

89

officials suggested that if a facility does not frequently serve as an originating site, it may not find it worthwhile to submit a claim for the approximately $25 originating site fee. Additionally, there may be cases where a beneficiary receives multiple telehealth services in a single day, and in such cases, the telehealth encounter might include several services that are appropriately billed with several claims from the distant site provider, but only have a single originating site claim.

However, according to MedPAC, the absence of originating site claims may have occurred because some patients may have inappropriately received services in their homes or other locations not permitted under the Medicare statute.[42] MedPAC also found that among the telehealth claims without corresponding originating site claims, 44 percent—or almost one-quarter of all telehealth claims made in calendar year 2014—were associated with beneficiaries living in urban areas, which could indicate that the patients were receiving telehealth services at inappropriate originating sites.[43] MedPAC officials told us that they identified one provider who conducted 2,000 telehealth visits in a single year, and all of those claims originated from an urban area.

When asked about MedPAC's findings, CMS officials told us that as of January 2017, they are reviewing the MedPAC report. They further stated that the agency will take action on MedPAC's findings, as warranted. This is consistent with federal standards for internal controls related to monitoring that call for managers to promptly evaluate findings from audits and other reviews—including those showing deficiencies—and determine and complete appropriate corrective actions.[44]

---

[42]Medicare has published information for providers to guide the use of telehealth. For example, in December 2015, CMS released a publication providing information on Medicare telehealth rules and regulations, including eligibility criteria for originating sites. In March 2016, CMS released guidance for providers submitting claims to the MACs for telehealth services provided to the beneficiaries. The guidance includes an address for a website that provides an updated list of Medicare telehealth services.

[43]MedPAC reported in 2013 that some physician practices billed errantly for telehealth services for urban patients because their billing managers were unaware of Medicare's location requirements for telehealth payment.

[44]GAO-14-704G, GAO/AIMD-00-21.3.1.

Selected Associations Report Telehealth and Remote Patient Monitoring May Improve Care for Medicare Beneficiaries, but Cited Coverage and Payment Restrictions as Barriers

Officials from selected associations representing providers and patients rated the significance of certain factors that encourage the use of telehealth and remote patient monitoring in Medicare as well as factors that create barriers to their use. The officials reported that both telehealth and remote patient monitoring may improve or maintain quality of care in Medicare, but they rated concerns regarding payment and coverage restrictions as potential barriers. Officials with a payer association we selected generally agreed with the assessments of the selected provider and patient associations.

Selected Associations Cited the Potential to Improve or Maintain Quality of Care as a Significant Factor Encouraging the Use of Telehealth and Remote Patient Monitoring in Medicare

Among the factors presented as potentially encouraging both telehealth and remote patient monitoring use in Medicare, officials from selected provider and patient associations most often rated the potential to improve or maintain quality of care as very or somewhat significant. (See fig. 2.) Officials from a provider association told us that telehealth can improve patient outcomes by facilitating follow-up to care. Additionally, an official from a patient association stated that remote patient monitoring is a helpful tool for treating patients with chronic disease.

Furthermore, officials from selected provider and patient associations more often rated alleviating provider shortages, convenience to patients, and coverage of services as very significant or somewhat significant factors that encourage both telehealth and remote patient monitoring use in Medicare. For example, officials from one provider association noted that provider and regional medical specialty shortages can be addressed through telehealth, potentially increasing productivity and ensuring on-time scheduling of appointments. Officials from another provider association reported that telehealth can increase convenience by shortening or eliminating travel times—which may lead to better adherence to recommended treatments and to patient satisfaction. Regarding remote patient monitoring, officials from a provider association explained that it can be an important tool for emergency department physicians to provide expertise to rural areas remotely, which could alleviate provider shortages.

Figure 2: Significance of Certain Factors That Encourage the Use of Telehealth and Remote Patient Monitoring in Medicare, According to Selected Provider and Patient Associations

Factor that encourages use	Provider associations						Patient associations	
	A	B	C	D	E	F	G	H
Improving or maintaining quality of care								
Telehealth	●	◐	●	●	◉	○	●	●
Remote patient monitoring	●	●	●	◉	●	◐	●	●
Alleviation of provider shortages/scheduling problems								
Telehealth	●	●	●	●	◉	●	◐	●
Remote patient monitoring	●	⊗	●	◉	●	⊗	●	●
Convenience for the patient								
Telehealth	◐	◐	●	●	◉	◐	●	●
Remote patient monitoring	◐	⊗	●	◉	●	◐	●	●
Coverage of services								
Telehealth	⊗	●	●	●	◉	●	◐	●
Remote patient monitoring	●	●	●	◉	●	⊗	◐	●

● A very significant factor that encourages use
◐ A somewhat significant factor that encourages use
○ A factor that encourages use, but not a significant one
⊗ Not a factor that encourages use
◉ Did not respond

Source: GAO analysis of a data collection instrument completed by six associations that represent providers and two associations that represent patients. | GAO-17-365

Note: Remote patient monitoring is a technology to enable monitoring of patients outside of conventional clinical settings, such as in the home.

Less frequently identified factors cited by association officials that encourage telehealth and remote patient monitoring use are described in the following examples, and in appendix V.

- Officials from two selected provider associations told us that emerging Medicare payment structures—such as accountable care

92

organizations (ACO)—could alleviate concerns about overutilization in Medicare's fee-for-service payment system.[45] The concern is that telehealth would be used in addition to, instead of in place of, face-to-face visits.

- Officials from one selected provider association stated that remote patient monitoring use shows promise in lowering health care costs and avoiding unneeded emergency room visits, because it allows a provider to identify subtle changes in a patient's condition and schedule an office visit before the patient's condition deteriorates.
- Officials from a selected patient association said that remote patient monitoring can help patients and their caregivers save on transportation costs and help them avoid having to miss work.

Although officials from the payer association we selected did not rate the significance of the factors, they confirmed that improving or maintaining quality of care was a factor in encouraging the use of both telehealth and remote patient monitoring. For example, officials stated that telehealth has the potential to decrease hospital readmissions and use of intensive care units. These officials also identified alleviating provider shortages and providing convenience for the patient as encouraging the use of telehealth. Additionally, these officials noted that the ability of patients to use their own electronic devices—such as home computers or smartphones—could facilitate broader use of remote patient monitoring services.

Selected Associations Cited Payment and Coverage Restrictions as Barriers to the Use of Telehealth and Remote Patient Monitoring in Medicare

Among the factors presented as potential barriers to the use of both telehealth and remote patient monitoring in Medicare, selected patient and provider associations most often rated cost increases or inadequate payment and coverage restrictions as very significant or somewhat significant. (See fig. 3.) Officials often linked their comments on payment with those regarding coverage restrictions. For example, officials from a provider association reported that Medicare's telehealth policies for payment and coverage lag behind other payers due to the program's statutory and regulatory restrictions. In particular, these restrictions limit the geographic and practice settings in which beneficiaries may receive

---

[45]ACOs are groups of physicians, hospitals, and other health care providers who voluntarily work together to give coordinated care to the Medicare patients they serve. See GAO, Medicare Value-Based Payment Models: Participation Challenges and Available Assistance for Small and Rural Practices, GAO-17-55 (Washington, D.C.: Dec. 9, 2016).

services, as well as the types of services that may be provided via telehealth and the types of technology that may be used.

Additionally, officials from another provider association described coverage as the single greatest barrier to the use of telehealth, adding that Medicare's restrictions on the types of services covered by the program have prohibited its broader use. Regarding remote patient monitoring, officials from another provider association stated that Medicare's valuation methodology for services results in low payment rates for remote patient monitoring, which these officials said remains a principal barrier to the use of these services. For more information on Medicare's valuation of remote patient monitoring, see appendix VI.

Officials from selected provider and patient associations more often rated infrastructure requirements as a very significant or somewhat significant barrier to the use of both telehealth and remote patient monitoring in Medicare. For example, officials from one provider association and both patient associations we selected described access to sufficiently reliable broadband internet service as a barrier to telehealth use. Officials from both of the patient associations also mentioned the ability to access the technology necessary to use telehealth as a potential barrier to its use. Officials from two of these provider associations also described uncertainty around which remote patient monitoring products and services are most effective.

94

Figure 3: Significance of Certain Barriers to the Use of Telehealth and Remote Patient Monitoring in Medicare, According to Selected Provider and Patient Associations

	Provider associations						Patient associations	
	A	B	C	D	E	F	G	H
Barrier to use								
Cost increase or inadequate payment								
Telehealth	●	●	⊗	●	●	●	⊗	●
Remote patient monitoring	●	●	●	●	●	◐	◐	●
Coverage of services								
Telehealth	●	●	○	●	●	●	●	●
Remote patient monitoring	●	●	●	●	●	◐	◐	●
Infrastructure Requirements								
Telehealth	◐	◐	⊗	◐	●	○	●	●
Remote patient monitoring	●	○	●	●	⊗	●	●	●

● A very significant barrier
◐ A somewhat significant barrier
○ A barrier, but not a significant one
⊗ Not a barrier
● Did not respond

Source: GAO analysis of a data collection instrument completed by six associations that represent providers and two associations that represent patients. | GAO-17-365

Note: Remote patient monitoring is a technology to enable monitoring of patients outside of conventional clinical settings, such as in the home.

Less frequently identified barriers to telehealth and remote patient monitoring use cited by selected provider and patient association officials are shown in the following examples, and in appendix V.

- Officials from both selected patient associations rated provider and patient training requirements as very significant barriers to the use of both telehealth and remote patient monitoring. Officials from one of these patient associations noted that training is important for patients, providers, and caregivers to help them understand the technology involved in using telehealth and remote patient monitoring.

- Officials from both selected patient associations also rated cultural factors, such as language and technological literacy, as very significant barriers to the use of both telehealth and remote patient monitoring.
- Officials from four selected provider associations rated professional licensure issues as a very or somewhat significant barrier to the use of telehealth. Officials from one association mentioned states' participation in the Interstate Medical Licensure Compact as a potential strategy to overcome telehealth licensure barriers.[46]

Although officials from the payer association we selected did not rate the significance of barriers to telehealth or remote patient monitoring use, they confirmed that cost increases and inadequate payment, as well as infrastructure requirements, are barriers to the use of these technologies. For example, officials cited as barriers equipment costs and the distribution of equipment to patients. Additionally, they discussed concerns about problems with the interoperability of platforms and devices used for telehealth.[47]

---

[46]The Interstate Medical Licensure Compact is a voluntary expedited pathway to licensure for physicians who wish to practice in multiple states.

[47]Interoperability is the ability of two or more systems or components to exchange information and to use the information that has been exchanged. See GAO, Electronic Health Records: DOD and VA Have Increased Their Sharing of Health Information, but More Work Remains, GAO-08-954 (Washington, D.C.: July 28, 2008).

CMS Has Various Efforts Underway That Have the Potential to Expand the Use of Telehealth and Remote Patient Monitoring in Medicare

CMS has efforts underway that have the potential to expand the use of telehealth and remote patient monitoring in Medicare. First, CMS supports models and demonstrations that offer alternative approaches to health care payment and delivery.[48] Second, CMS's new Medicare payment program allows participating clinicians to use telehealth, and to some extent remote patient monitoring, to help them achieve some of the goals of the payment program.[49]

CMS Models and Demonstrations

The Patient Protection and Affordable Care Act created the Innovation Center within CMS to test innovative payment and service delivery models to reduce Medicare, Medicaid, and state Children's Health Insurance Program expenditures while preserving or enhancing the quality of care for beneficiaries of the programs.[50] The Innovation Center also supports Medicare demonstration projects, which study the likely impact of new methods of service delivery, coverage of new types of services, and new payment approaches on beneficiaries, providers, health plans, states, and the Medicare trust funds. The Innovation Center has the authority to waive Medicare telehealth requirements as part of its efforts to implement and test these models and, as allowed by other statutory authorities, as part of testing demonstrations.

---

[48]Models are new payment and service delivery structures developed by CMS under the authority of section 1115A of the Social Security Act. Demonstration projects study the likely impact of new methods of service delivery, coverage of new types of services, and new payment approaches on beneficiaries, providers, health plans, states, and the Medicare trust funds. These demonstration projects are established under other statutory authorities.

[49]The Merit-based Incentive Payment System applies to eligible clinicians, defined as physicians, physician assistants, nurse practitioners, clinical nurse specialists, certified registered nurse anesthetists, and groups that include such clinicians who bill under Medicare Part B. While we refer to "providers" elsewhere in our report, we use the term "clinicians" when discussing the Merit-based Incentive Payment System.

[50]Pub. L. No. 111-148, §§ 3021, 10306, 124 Stat. 119, 389, 939 (codified at 42 U.S.C. § 1315a).

According to CMS, telehealth waivers may broaden access to telehealth services, and CMS's Innovation Center has used its authority, and other statutory authorities as applicable, to waive Medicare telehealth requirements for eight models and demonstrations in certain circumstances.[51] Specifically, CMS's Innovation Center waived certain requirements regarding the geographic location or types of permitted sites at which beneficiaries can receive telehealth services for four models:

- Next Generation ACOs are groups of doctors, hospitals, and other health care providers and suppliers who come together voluntarily to provide coordinated, high-quality care at lower costs to their Medicare patients.[52]
- Two Bundled Payments for Care Improvement models link payments for the multiple services beneficiaries receive during an episode of care.[53] Under this initiative, organizations enter into payment arrangements that include financial and performance accountability for episodes of care.
- The Comprehensive Care for Joint Replacement Model aims to support better and more efficient care for beneficiaries undergoing hip and knee replacements, which are the most common inpatient surgeries for Medicare beneficiaries.[54]

Additionally, CMS officials told us that three Episode Payment Models will have telehealth waivers removing Medicare's geographic and permitted site telehealth requirements beginning sometime in calendar year 2017 and will pay providers for care based on the following conditions treated:

- acute myocardial infarction,

---

[51] The Social Security Act provides authority for the Secretary of Health and Human Services to waive Medicare payment requirements as may be necessary for the Innovation Center to test payment and delivery service models. According to CMS officials, the statutory authorities of certain demonstrations have provided similar authority to waive Medicare telehealth requirements.

[52] As of January 2017, there were 45 Next Generation ACO model participants.

[53] When we refer to the Bundled Payments for Care Improvement Model, we are referring to model two, Retrospective Acute & Post Acute Care Episode, and model three, Retrospective Post Acute Care Only, which are the two Bundled Payments for Care Improvement models with access to the telehealth waiver. As of January 2017, model two has 577 participants and model three has 779 participants.

[54] Comprehensive Care for Joint Replacement Model participation is required in 67 Metropolitan Statistical Areas.

- coronary artery bypass grafts, and
- surgical hip and femur fractures.[55]

Furthermore, in one demonstration that aims to develop and test new models of integrated health care in sparsely populated rural counties—the Frontier Community Health Integration Project Demonstration—CMS allows participants to receive cost-based payments for telehealth when their location serves as the originating site, rather than the approximately $25 fixed fee that CMS otherwise pays originating sites.[56] See table 2 for more information on the Medicare telehealth requirements waived for these models and demonstrations.

CMS officials told us that the Innovation Center also has the authority to waive requirements regarding payment for telehealth services for payment and delivery service models, but that the Innovation Center identified waiving requirements regarding the originating site as the best way to provide broader access to telehealth.[57] The Innovation Center could potentially waive other telehealth requirements if it decided to do so in the future.

---

[55] According to CMS officials, the Acute Myocardial Infarction Model and the Coronary Artery Bypass Graft Model will be implemented in 98 Metropolitan Statistical Areas, accounting for approximately 1,127 hospitals, and the Surgical Hip and Femur Fracture Treatment Model will be implemented in the 67 Metropolitan Statistical Areas where the Comprehensive Care for Joint Replacement Model is also occurring, accounting for 866 hospitals.

[56] The Frontier Community Health Integration Project Demonstration has 10 rural health care participants, and of those, 8 have telehealth as a demonstration intervention tool. CMS officials told us that CMS initially explored implementing a store-and-forward waiver for this demonstration, which would have allowed providers to, for example, take a photo of a skin condition, then send that photo to a dermatologist at a distant site for review. CMS officials told us they determined that it was not operationally feasible to implement that waiver within the demonstration period.

[57] CMS officials told us that CMS also has the authority to waive some telehealth requirements for other demonstration projects through other statutory authority.

Table 2: Medicare Telehealth Requirements Waived for Selected Models and Demonstrations

Requirement	Change in Medicare telehealth requirement under waiver	Applicable models and demonstrations
Originating site geography	This waiver removes the requirement that telehealth only occur in • a rural health professional shortage area, • a county that is not included in a Metropolitan Statistical Area, or • an entity that participates in a federal telehealth demonstration project (referred to as telemedicine demonstration projects in statute) approved by or receiving funding from the Secretary of Health and Human Services as of December 31, 2000.	Bundled Payments for Care Improvement Model[a] Comprehensive Care for Joint Replacement Model Episode Payment Models[b] Next Generation Accountable Care Organizations
Originating site type	The waiver allows for telehealth services to be furnished in the patient's home or place of residence and eliminates the requirement that the patient receiving telehealth services must be at one of the specified originating sites: • physician or provider office, • critical access hospital, • rural health clinic, • federally qualified health center, • hospital, • hospital-based or critical access hospital-based renal dialysis center or satellites, • skilled nursing facility, or • community mental health center. The waiver eliminates the requirement to pay originating site fees when telehealth services are provided in the patient's home.	Comprehensive Care for Joint Replacement Model Episode Payment Models[b] Next Generation Accountable Care Organizations
Originating site facility fee	The waiver allows participants to receive cost-based payment for telehealth when they are the originating site, rather than the approximately $25 set fee for originating sites.	Frontier Community Health Integration Project Demonstration

Source: GAO analysis of Medicare statute and Centers for Medicare & Medicaid Services (CMS) regulations. | GAO-17-365

Note: The term "originating site" refers to the location where the patient is located while receiving a telehealth service.

[a]The Bundled Payments for Care Improvement Model refers in this case only to Bundled Payments for Care Improvement models two and three.

[b]Episode Payment Models refer to three models for episodes of care surrounding (1) acute myocardial infarction, (2) coronary artery bypass graft, and (3) surgical hip/femur fracture treatment. CMS officials told us that these models would begin sometime in calendar year 2017.

In calendar year 2015, 15 Next Generation ACOs submitted implementation plans that detailed their proposed strategies to implement the telehealth waiver.[58] Eleven out of the 15 expected to use telehealth to provide increased access to specialty providers.[59] For example, one participant reported that it would use telehealth to establish a virtual network of specialists who could provide telehealth consultations to patients in areas such as cardiology, rheumatology, and psychiatry. In addition, 8 out of 15 Next Generation ACOs included plans to use telehealth to improve care for patients with chronic conditions.[60] For example, one participant planned to use telehealth to connect beneficiaries who have chronic diseases—such as congestive heart failure, diabetes, and pulmonary diseases—with their care team, including specialty providers.

As table 3 shows, the Innovation Center models and demonstration with waivers are in various stages of implementation, and their participants are using telehealth to varying degrees.

---

[58] There were 18 Next Generation ACOs operating in calendar year 2016, and of those, 15 provided CMS with implementation plans to use telehealth waivers. CMS officials told us that implementation plans were also required for the Frontier Community Health Integration Project Demonstration, but not for the other models with telehealth waivers.

[59] The remaining four Next Generation ACOs may plan to provide increased access to specialty providers through the use of telehealth; however, their implementation plans did not explicitly state that this was the ACOs' intent under the waiver.

[60] The remaining seven Next Generation ACOs may plan to use telehealth to improve care for patients with chronic conditions; however, their implementation plans did not explicitly state that this was the ACOs' intent under the waiver.

Table 3: Telehealth Use by Selected Models and Demonstrations with Waivers of Certain Medicare Requirements

Model or demonstration	Time period of services	Number of Medicare telehealth services provided	Additional information
Bundled Payments for Care Improvement Model[a]	October 2013-June 2015	7	CMS officials told us that during this period model participants performed a total of 166,000 services.
Next Generation Accountable Care Organization (ACO) Model	January 2016-June 2016	1,422	According to CMS officials, telehealth services were concentrated among a few ACOs. One ACO accounted for more than half of all the telehealth claims, and five each had more than 50 telehealth claims. CMS officials said that around one-third of the telehealth services provided were for beneficiaries residing in urban areas, and the officials said they could attribute this use to the waiver.
Comprehensive Care for Joint Replacement Model	April 2016-September 2016	0	CMS officials said that as of January 2017 these data were still preliminary and may not include all claims for care that occurred between April 2016 and September 2016. As a result, there may be claims for telehealth services delivered as part of the Comprehensive Care for Joint Replacement Model during that time frame that are not yet reflected in CMS's claims data.
Frontier Community Health Integration Project Demonstration	n/a	n/a	CMS officials told us that as of January 2017, they did not have data on the utilization of the originating site facility fee waiver, as the demonstration has only been operational for a few months.
Episode Payment Model[b]	n/a	n/a	CMS officials told us that these models would begin sometime in calendar year 2017.

Source: GAO analysis of Centers for Medicare & Medicaid Services (CMS) reports and interviews. | GAO-17-365

Note: n/a = not applicable.

[a]The Bundled Payments for Care Improvement Model refers in this case only to Bundled Payments for Care Improvement models two and three.

[b]Episode Payment Models refer to three models for episodes of care surrounding (1) acute myocardial infarction, (2) coronary artery bypass graft, and (3) surgical hip/femur fracture treatment.

In addition to the models and demonstrations in which CMS waives certain telehealth requirements, other models and demonstrations may affect the use of telehealth, as described in the following examples.

- Under its Health Care Innovation Award program, CMS funds cooperative agreements that the agency identifies as the most compelling new ideas to deliver better health, improve care, and lower

102

costs to Medicare, Medicaid, and state Children's Health Insurance Program beneficiaries.[61] Some of these projects include initiatives focused on telehealth and remote patient monitoring.[62] For example, one award supported efforts to use telehealth and remote patient monitoring to provide care for urban and rural Medicare patients receiving intensive care. An evaluation of this awardee found the effort was associated with a reduction in hospital readmissions.[63]

- According to CMS documents, in the Initiative to Reduce Avoidable Hospitalizations among Nursing Facility Residents—which aims to improve the quality of care for individuals residing in long-term care facilities by reducing avoidable hospitalizations—a participant plans to use telehealth to evaluate nursing home residents whose conditions worsen at night when physicians are not present.[64]

- The Independence at Home Demonstration, which tests a payment incentive and service delivery model that uses primary care teams to provide in-home primary care to Medicare beneficiaries with multiple chronic conditions, includes practices that have the ability to use remote monitoring and mobile diagnostic technology with their patients.[65]

For more examples of how telehealth and remote patient monitoring may be used in models and demonstrations, see appendix VII.

---

[61] A cooperative agreement is a legal instrument used to provide financial support when substantial interaction is expected between a federal agency and a state, local government, or other recipient carrying out the funded activity.

[62] Round one of the Health Care Innovation Awards funded up to $1 billion in awards over three years through cooperative agreements. A 2015 CMS report shows that 17 of the agency's 108 round one Health Care Innovation Awards include a telehealth or remote patient monitoring component. Department of Health and Human Services, Center for Medicare & Medicaid Innovation, Health Care Innovation Awards (HCIA) Meta-Analysis and Evaluators Collaborative, Annual Report Year 1.

[63] Round two of the Health Care Innovation Awards funded up to $360 million in awards. CMS officials told us that of the 39 round two Health Care Innovation Awards, 7 focused on telehealth. The officials told us the awards were underway and that evaluation results are not yet available.

[64] As of January 2017, there were seven organizations selected for the Initiative to Reduce Avoidable Hospitalizations among Nursing Facility Residents.

[65] This demonstration supports home-based primary care for Medicare beneficiaries with multiple chronic conditions.

103

Merit-based Incentive Payment System	Beginning in 2017, CMS will implement the Quality Payment Program, which will include a new Medicare payment program—the Merit-based Incentive Payment System—for physicians and other clinicians. The Merit-based Incentive Payment System will consolidate components of programs currently used to tie payments to quality and provide incentives for quality, resource use, clinical practice improvement activities, and advancing care information through the meaningful use of electronic health record technology.[66] Under this payment program, clinicians can use telehealth in certain ways to meet the criteria in the program's improvement activities performance category, which can help clinicians improve their performance under the payment program.[67] For example, clinicians could use telehealth to coordinate care and, in some cases, to reach patients in remote locations. Additionally, there are some instances when clinicians can use remote patient monitoring to meet Merit-based Incentive Payment System goals—for example, using home monitoring to remotely gather information to determine a patient's proper dose of blood thinning medication. According to CMS officials, clinicians using telehealth and remote patient monitoring for these purposes do not have to bill Medicare for the service in order to receive credit for it under the Merit-based Incentive Payment System, and these services can count for credit under the improvement activities performance category regardless of whether they meet the statutory telehealth requirements. However, if clinicians want to bill Medicare for these services, the service must meet Medicare's statutory requirements for payment.
Agency and Third-Party Comments	We provided a draft of this report to HHS, DOD, and VA for review and comment. These departments provided technical comments, which we incorporated as appropriate. We also provided relevant draft portions of this report to stakeholders we interviewed. Specifically, we provided these excerpts to state Medicaid program officials for Connecticut, Illinois, Kansas, Mississippi, Montana,

---

[66] 81 Fed. Reg. 77010. Components of the previously separate Physician Quality Reporting System, Physician Value-based Payment Modifier program, and Medicare electronic health record incentive program will be merged into the Merit-based Incentive Payment System so that payments for most physicians will reflect physician performance on both quality measures and electronic health record use. See GAO-17-55.

[67] Improvement activities are those that support broad aims within health care delivery, including care coordination, beneficiary engagement, population management, and health equity.

and Oregon; representatives of selected provider, patient, and payer associations; and officials from selected private payers. Not all of the stakeholders responded. One state and one association confirmed that the information we provided was accurate. In addition, three states, four associations, and three private payers provided technical comments, which we incorporated as appropriate.

We are sending copies of this report to the appropriate congressional committees, the Secretary of Health and Human Services, Secretary of the Department of Defense, Secretary of the Department of Veterans Affairs, and to other interested parties. In addition, the report is available at no charge on the GAO website at http://www.gao.gov.

If you or your staff have any questions about this report, please contact me at (202) 512-7114 or YocomC@gao.gov. Contact points for our Offices of Congressional Relations and Public Affairs may be found on the last page of this report. GAO staff who made key contributions to this report are listed in appendix VIII.

Carolyn L. Yocom
Director, Health Care

List of Requesters

The Honorable Orrin Hatch
Chairman
The Honorable Ron Wyden
Ranking Member
Committee on Finance
United States Senate

The Honorable Lamar Alexander
Chairman
The Honorable Patty Murray
Ranking Member
Committee on Health, Education, Labor, and Pensions
United States Senate

The Honorable Greg Walden
Chairman
The Honorable Frank Pallone
Ranking Member
Committee on Energy and Commerce
House of Representatives

The Honorable Kevin Brady
Chairman
The Honorable Richard Neal
Ranking Member
Committee on Ways and Means
House of Representatives

Appendix I: Use of Remote Patient Monitoring by Selected Private Payers

As part of our work, we interviewed officials from health plans in the private insurance market (private payers) about the use of remote patient monitoring.[1] This appendix provides the results of those interviews. Officials from three of the top private payers (based on market share) told us that providers can use remote patient monitoring in their health care systems when it is indicated for a patient's condition.[2]

Officials from the three private payers told us they have limited data on the extent to which remote patient monitoring is used. They told us they did not have data available because, for example, remote patient monitoring services are usually part of a care management program in which charges are bundled and not billed and detailed separately. It is therefore difficult to distinguish remote patient monitoring services from services provided via telehealth, officials explained. Some of the health plans of these three private payers reimburse for remote patient monitoring on a fee-for-service basis, while others include it as part of the services offered through integrated delivery systems that do not reimburse for separate services.

Officials from one private payer explained that they want physicians to decide which patients, conditions, problems, and circumstances are most suited to remote patient monitoring. This private payer does not reimburse physicians on a fee-for-service basis, noting that incentives, such as payment, can drive behavior. As an example, if the provider receives reimbursement based on the amount of monitoring, the provider may file more claims for monitoring, regardless of whether the use is driven by evidence-based care processes. Instead, officials from this private payer stated that their incentives focus on the care outcomes of physicians' patients, and they pay physicians based on the quality of the outcomes by disease population. Officials explained that they are currently rolling out programs to track diabetic patients' blood sugar by monitoring what they eat, the exercise they get, and how they live. Additionally, this private payer has been using remote patient monitoring for patients with heart failure for some time, and officials told us that data

---

[1] Remote patient monitoring is a technology to enable monitoring of patients outside of conventional clinical settings, such as the home.

[2] The three private payers we interviewed were in the top five payers by market share in the accident and health insurance industry based on the National Association of Insurance Commissioners' 2015 report. See National Association of Insurance Commissioners, 2014 Market Share Reports: For the Top 125 Accident and Health Insurance Groups and Companies by State and Countrywide (2015).

Appendix I: Use of Remote Patient Monitoring by Selected Private Payers

gathered through monitoring of weight and blood pressure are good predictors of early deterioration of heart conditions. Similarly, this private payer has a program for patients with hypertension that monitors a patient's stress level.

Officials from a second private payer stated that they reimburse for remote patient monitoring in a manner that is appropriate for the specific condition being treated. For example, they reimburse for cardiologic remote patient monitoring if the patient has symptoms that are indications for the use of monitoring. If the condition does not indicate cardiologic monitoring, the private payer does not reimburse for this monitoring. Officials from this second private payer said they are reimbursing for remote patient monitoring that is used in real time to monitor patients with one or more chronic conditions and for high-risk patients. For example, the service is used to monitor blood pressure for hypertension, weight changes for congestive heart failure, and real-time blood sugar for diabetes. According to these private payer officials, providers typically use remote patient monitoring in the short-term and episodically, or to retrospectively look at monitoring results to make a clinical decision. Remote patient monitoring is also used to connect health plan members with their care managers, and these managers can notify providers to intervene if the monitoring indicates a need. This private payer also has various pilot programs related to remote patient monitoring, including a program for its members with varying levels of congestive heart failure.

Officials from the third private payer told us that if remote patient monitoring is indicated by a patient's condition, then the provider can order its use. Some of the payer's private plans are integrated delivery systems for overall care, and in these plans providers are not paid separately for remote patient monitoring. According to officials, their agreements with providers are designed to encourage providers to use data from all sources, such as claims information, electronic medical records, and remote patient monitoring. The private payer also contracts with accountable care organizations and enters into payment arrangements with provider groups.[3] Those entities use remote patient monitoring and the information obtained through monitoring as part of their care management of patients. This private payer's fee-for-service

---

[3]Accountable care organizations are groups of physicians, hospitals, and other health care providers who voluntarily work together to provide coordinated care to the Medicare patients they serve.

109

Appendix I: Use of Remote Patient Monitoring by Selected Private Payers

plans reimburse for remote patient monitoring services, including cardiac services.

Officials from all three private payers told us that there are challenges to using remote patient monitoring in the private sector. For example, officials from one private payer said that barriers to the use of remote patient monitoring can include the need to set up equipment in the patient's home, interact with members with cognitive and physical disabilities and their caregivers, and address technical difficulties with the equipment.

Appendix II: Scope and Methodology for Identifying Factors Affecting the Use of Telehealth and Remote Patient Monitoring

We administered a data collection instrument to selected associations representing providers, patients, and payers to obtain information on the factors that encourage the use of telehealth and remote patient monitoring in Medicare or are barriers to their use. To develop the data collection instrument, we identified a list of potential factors and barriers based on background research and initial interviews with two groups with an interest in telehealth. Table 4 displays the list of factors that encourage use or are barriers to use as they appeared in the data collection instrument.[1] For the purposes of the data collection instrument, we defined telehealth as clinical services that are provided remotely via telecommunications technologies, and we defined remote patient monitoring as a technology to enable monitoring of patients outside of conventional clinical settings, such as in the home.

Table 4: Potential Factors that Encourage the Use or Are Barriers to the Use of Telehealth or Remote Patient Monitoring in Medicare Used in the Data Collection Instrument

Potential factors that encourage or are barriers[a]	If Yes, how significant is the factor that encourages or is a barrier?			
	Is this a factor that encourages or is a barrier (Y/N)?	Not Significant	Somewhat Significant	Very Significant
Factors that encourage use				
Alleviation of provider shortages/scheduling problems				
Convenience for the patient				
Cost reduction				
Coverage of services				
Emerging Medicare payment structures or waivers				
Enabling the use of emerging technology				
Health Resources and Services Administration telehealth grant programs/other federal initiatives				
Improving or maintaining quality of care				
Other: please list any other factors				
Barriers to use				
Concern regarding quality of care				

[1]For the purposes of this report, we combined the tables for factors that encourage use or are barriers to use in one table. In the data collection instrument, the factors that encourage use or are barriers to use were separate for both telehealth and remote patient monitoring.

Appendix II: Scope and Methodology for Identifying Factors Affecting the Use of Telehealth and Remote Patient Monitoring

Cost increase or inadequate payment
Coverage of services
Cultural factors[b]
Infrastructure requirements[c]
Pace of changing technology
Privacy and security concerns
Professional licensure issues
Provider/patient training requirements
Other: please list any other barriers

Source: GAO analysis of background research documents and interviews with two groups with an interest in telehealth. | GAO-17-365

Note: Remote patient monitoring is a technology to enable monitoring of patients outside of conventional clinical settings, such as in the home.

[a]We used the word "incentive" in the data collection instrument, which we are referring to as "factors that encourage" for the purpose of our report.

[b]Cultural factors may include language and technological literacy, among others.

[c]Infrastructure requirements may include access to broadband internet, imaging technology or peripherals, and wireless communications systems, among others.

To identify associations that might have an interest in telehealth and remote patient monitoring, we conducted background research, interviewed two groups with an interest in telehealth, and used knowledge from our previous engagements to judgmentally select associations based on their relevance and expertise. We chose associations that represented three health care perspectives—providers, patients, and payers. In addition, we chose medical specialty associations that represent common conditions for which telehealth or remote patient monitoring may be used, or could be beneficial, during the course of treatment, such as stroke, heart disease and congestive heart failure, and mental health. We included nine associations in our review: six associations that represent providers, two associations that represent patients, and one association representing payers.[2]

A representative of the payer association we spoke with told us that it did not have sufficient time to survey its members and could not complete our data collection instrument without doing so. Therefore, we reported

[2]These associations are AARP, America's Health Insurance Plans, American Heart Association/American Stroke Association, American Hospital Association, American Medical Association, American Telemedicine Association, National Association of Rural Health Clinics, National Patient Advocate Foundation, and Remote Cardiac Services Provider Group.

Appendix II: Scope and Methodology for Identifying Factors Affecting the Use of Telehealth and Remote Patient Monitoring

separately the payer association's views on factors that encourage the use of, or are barriers to, telehealth and remote patient monitoring. For the payer association, we interviewed officials to identify factors that encourage use or are barriers to the use of telehealth and remote patient monitoring in Medicare. We used professional judgment based on information obtained throughout the course of our engagement to match the payer association officials' statements on factors that encourage use or are barriers to use with corresponding data collection instrument factors that encourage use or are barriers to use.

After identifying the associations, we administered the data collection instrument and requested that officials from each association rate each factor that encourages the use of telehealth and remote patient monitoring and each barrier to use. We requested that officials rate factors that encourage telehealth use, factors that encourage remote patient monitoring use, barriers to telehealth use, and barriers to remote patient monitoring use. For example, if an official identified a factor as encouraging the use of telehealth, we requested that the official rate the factor as not significant, somewhat significant, or very significant.

To identify the factors that encourage use or are barriers to use that were rated either most often or more often "very significant" or "somewhat significant" by the associations who completed our data collection instrument, we developed the following scoring system.

- Highest points (5) were assigned to an individual factor when an association rated it very significant for both telehealth and remote patient monitoring.
- Next highest points (3) were assigned to an individual factor when an association rated it very significant for either telehealth or remote patient monitoring and somewhat significant for either telehealth or remote patient monitoring.
- Lowest points (1) were assigned to an individual factor when an association rated it somewhat significant for both telehealth and remote patient monitoring.

No points were assigned for any other rating combinations.

We used this scoring system to separately calculate total points assigned to (1) each individual factor that encouraged use, and (2) each factor considered to be a barrier to use. Within either group (either among those that encouraged use or among those that were considered barriers to use), if any one or two factors had measurably greater scores than the

Appendix II: Scope and Methodology for Identifying Factors Affecting the Use of Telehealth and Remote Patient Monitoring

other factors, those factors were reported as rated most often very significant or somewhat significant. Additionally, we determined whether any other factor or several factors had obviously higher scores than the remaining factors that either encourage use or are a barrier to use, and we reported those factors as rated more often very significant or somewhat significant.

We also interviewed officials from each association using a structured question set to obtain examples of how these factors can encourage or create barriers to the use of telehealth and remote patient monitoring in Medicare. Finally, we obtained and reviewed any relevant documentation from these associations. The perspectives we obtained using the data collection instrument, from our document reviews, and during our interviews with association officials provided insights regarding officials' views about the factors that encourage the use of telehealth and remote patient monitoring and the factors that are barriers to their use. These perspectives cannot be generalized to other associations or officials.

Appendix III: Medicare Telehealth Services Added and Denied by the Centers for Medicare & Medicaid Services, 2011-2016

The Centers for Medicare & Medicaid Service (CMS)—an agency within the Department of Health and Human Services—has a process for adding or denying proposed services to the list of Medicare telehealth services.[1] This process provides the public with an ongoing opportunity to submit requests for adding services. Under this process, CMS assigns requests to one of two categories:

1. services that are similar to professional consultations, office visits, and office psychiatry services that are currently on the list of telehealth services; and

2. services that are not similar to the current list of telehealth services. In reviewing these requests, CMS looks for evidence indicating that the use of a telecommunications system in furnishing the requested telehealth service produces clinical benefit for the patient.

The most common reason a proposed service was added for payment from calendar years 2011 through 2016 was similarity to a service already on the list of telehealth services. See table 5 for the Current Procedural Terminology and Healthcare Common Procedure Coding System codes that were approved by CMS, including the reason for adding the service, from calendar year 2011 through calendar year 2016.

---

[1] Medicare pays for a limited number of Part B services furnished by a physician or provider to an eligible beneficiary via a telecommunications system. Part B services include physician and outpatient hospital services. For eligible telehealth services, the use of a telecommunications system substitutes for an in-person encounter.

Appendix III: Medicare Telehealth Services Added and Denied by the Centers for Medicare & Medicaid Services, 2011-2016

Table 5: Telehealth Service Codes Added by the Centers for Medicare & Medicaid Services (CMS), Calendar Years 2011 through 2016

Calendar year	Service code	Description of service	CMS rationale for adding the service
2011	G0108 G0109	Individual and group diabetes outpatient self-management training services	CMS initially denied this in 2009 because it might involve injection training. The agency approved it as sufficiently similar to G0270 medical nutrition therapy, but requires 1 hour of in-person injection training.
	G0420 G0421	Individual and group kidney disease education	Similar to another telehealth code, G0270 medical nutrition therapy.
	96153 96154 97804	Group medical nutrition therapy services, and group Health Behavior Assessment and Intervention services	Similar to other telehealth codes.
	99231 99232 99233	Subsequent hospital care services	Similar to follow-up inpatient consultation services. These services can only be furnished through telehealth once every 3 days.
	99307 99308 99309 99310	Subsequent nursing facility care services	Similar to other telehealth codes. These services can only be furnished through telehealth once every 30 days.
2012	99406 99407 G0436 G0437	Smoking and tobacco use cessation counseling, intermediate and intensive	Similar to individual kidney disease education reported by code G0420 and individual medical nutrition therapy services reported by G0270, 97802, and 97803.
2013	G0396 G0397	Alcohol and substance abuse assessment, 15 to 30 minutes and greater than 30 minutes, respectively	Similar to an existing telehealth service: smoking cessation counseling 99406 and 99407.
	G0442 G0443 G0444 G0445 G0446 G0447	Screening for behavioral conditions: alcohol misuse and counseling, depression, sexually transmitted infections, cardiovascular disease, and obesity	Similar to existing behavioral intervention telehealth codes.
2014	99495 99496	Transitional care management services with follow up communication, 14 days and 7 days after discharge, respectively	Similar to other telehealth services.
2015	G0438 G0439	Annual wellness visit, initial and subsequent, respectively	Similar to existing behavioral intervention telehealth codes.
	90845 90846 90847	Psychoanalysis, family psychotherapy without patient, and family psychotherapy with patient, respectively	Similar to existing behavioral intervention telehealth codes.
	99354 99355	Prolonged service in the office or other outpatient setting requiring direct patient contact beyond the usual service, first hour and each additional 30 minutes, respectively	Similar to existing behavioral intervention telehealth codes.

Appendix III: Medicare Telehealth Services Added and Denied by the Centers for Medicare & Medicaid Services, 2011-2016

Calendar year	Service code	Description of service	CMS rationale for adding the service
2016	90963 90964 90965 90966	End-stage renal disease related services for home dialysis per full month; patients younger than ages 2, 2-11, 12-19, and 20+, respectively	Similar to existing psychiatric diagnostic procedures or office/outpatient visits codes.
	99356 99357	Prolonged service in the inpatient or observation settings, requiring unit/floor time beyond the usual service; first hour and additional 30 minutes, respectively	Similar to existing psychiatric diagnostic procedures or office/outpatient visits codes.

Source: GAO analysis of Federal Register Notices for Medicare Telehealth Services. | GAO-17-365

There are several reasons that CMS denied proposed services for its approved telehealth list for calendar years 2011 through 2016. These reasons are, for example, that

- the service was not like any other on the telehealth list, and the requester could not prove to CMS that the service is effective when furnished through telehealth;
- the service was furnished by a provider or in a location that is not allowed under Medicare;
- the service was not face-to-face when not provided via telehealth; and
- the service required face-to-face care because of patient acuity or another factor.

See table 6 for the Current Procedural Terminology and Healthcare Common Procedure Coding System codes that were denied by CMS and the reasons for denial, from calendar year 2011 through calendar year 2016.

Appendix III: Medicare Telehealth Services Added and Denied by the Centers for Medicare & Medicaid Services, 2011-2016

Table 6: Telehealth Service Codes Denied by the Centers for Medicare & Medicaid Services (CMS), Calendar Years 2011 through 2016

Calendar year	Service code	Description of service	CMS rationale for denial
2011	96119	Neuropsychological testing	Not similar to other telehealth services; no studies were provided on the efficacy of this service when provided through telehealth.
	99221 99222 99223	Level 1, 2, and 3 initial hospital care, respectively	No current telehealth codes resemble initial hospital care like these, and CMS was not convinced by studies provided in support of the request.
	99238 99239	Hospital discharge management, less than 30 minutes and more, respectively	There are no services on the current list of telehealth services that resemble such preparation of a patient for discharge. CMS was not convinced by the studies provided in support of the request.
	99304 99305 99306 99315 99316 99318	Nursing facility care codes—initial, discharge, and annual assessment	Codes 99304, 99305, 99306, and 99318 are federally-mandated nursing facility visits that should be provided in person. Codes 99315 and 99316 are not required to be furnished under Medicare, but if a provider chooses to provide these services, the services should be provided in person. No current telehealth codes resemble this preparation of a patient for discharge, and CMS did not have evidence that these services provided via telehealth are equivalent to in-person services.
	No code provided	Home wound care	The home is not an eligible telehealth originating site under Medicare.
	No code provided	Speech language pathology services	Speech language pathologists are not eligible telehealth providers under Medicare.
2012	96040	Medical genetics and genetic counseling services	The services under this code would only be furnished by genetics counselors, who are not eligible telehealth providers.
	99090 99091	Analysis of clinical data stored in computers and collection and interpretation of physiologic data	As explained in a 2002 final rule, this code is part of pre- and post-work for a separate and unspecified evaluation and management code. These codes are not separately payable. CMS also denied these codes in 2015.
	99291 99292	Critical care, evaluation and management of the critically ill or critically injured patient, first 30 to 74 minutes and each additional 30 minutes, respectively	Previously considered and denied adding these codes in 2009 and 2010 because critical care services are not similar to any services on the current list of Medicare telehealth services and CMS believes patients requiring critical care services are more acutely ill than typical patients receiving telehealth services. Additionally, CMS did not have evidence that these services provided via telehealth are equivalent to in-person services.
	99334 99335 99336 99337	Domiciliary or rest home evaluation and management visit; 15 minute visit, 25 minute visit, 40 minute visit, and 60 minute visit respectively	A domiciliary or rest home is not an eligible telehealth originating site under Medicare.
	99444	Online evaluation and management	As indicated in 2008, 2012, 2014, and 2016, this is a noncovered service because it is non-face-to-face and the language of the descriptor indicates that the service could be for noncovered entities, like guardians.

Appendix III: Medicare Telehealth Services Added and Denied by the Centers for Medicare & Medicaid Services, 2011-2016

Calendar year	Service code	Description of service	CMS rationale for denial
	No code provided	Audiology services	Audiologists are not authorized telehealth providers under Medicare.
2013	99408 99409	Alcohol and substance abuse screening, 15 to 30 minutes and greater than 30 minutes, respectively	These are noncovered services under the Physician Fee Schedule.[a] As explained in 2008, Medicare only provides payment for certain screening services with an explicit benefit category. However, CMS created parallel codes—G0396 and G0397—and approved those for the telehealth list.
2014	98969	Online assessment and management service provided by a non-physician	These are noncovered services because it is non-face-to-face and the language of the descriptor indicates that the service could be for noncovered entities, like guardians.
	99444	Online evaluation and management	As indicated in comments for 2008, 2012, 2014, and 2016, this is a noncovered service because it is non-face-to-face and the language of the descriptor indicates that the service could be for noncovered entities, like guardians.
2015	57452 57454 57460	Colposcopy of the cervix, colposcopy of the cervix with biopsy, and colposcopy of the cervix with loop electrode biopsy(s) of the cervix, respectively	These services are not similar to other services on the telehealth list and the requester did not submit evidence to support the clinical benefit of furnishing these services via telehealth.
	90887 99090 99091 99358 99359	Interpretation of psychiatric examinations, analysis of clinical data stored in computers, collection and interpretation of physiologic data, prolonged evaluation and management, first hour and each additional 30 minutes, respectively	Medicare does not make a separate payment for these services.
	92250 93010 93307 93308 93320 93321 93325	Fundus photography with interpretation and report, and five types of echocardiography services	These services include a technical component and a professional component. By definition, the technical component portion of these services needs to be furnished in the same location as the patient and thus cannot be furnished via telehealth.
	96103 96120	Psychological testing, neuropsychological testing, respectively	These services involve testing by computer, can be furnished remotely without the patient being present, and are payable in the same way as other physicians' services. These services are not Medicare telehealth services.
	96101 96102 96118 96119	Psychological testing per hour of physician time and technician time; neuropsychological testing per hour of physician time and technician time, respectively	These services are not similar to other services on the telehealth list, as they require close observation of how a patient responds. The requester did not submit evidence supporting the clinical benefit of furnishing these services via telehealth.
	No code provided	Urgent dermatologic problems and wound care	Without a specified code, CMS cannot determine if this is an appropriate telehealth service.

Appendix III: Medicare Telehealth Services Added and Denied by the Centers for Medicare & Medicaid Services, 2011-2016

Calendar year	Service code	Description of service	CMS rationale for denial
2016	99291 99292	Critical care, evaluation and management of the critically ill or critically injured patient, first 30 to 74 minutes and each additional 30 minutes, respectively	Previously considered and denied adding these codes in 2009, 2010, and 2012 because critical care services are not similar to any services on the current list of Medicare telehealth services, and CMS believes patients requiring critical care services are more acutely ill than typical patients receiving telehealth services. Additionally, CMS did not have evidence that these services provided via telehealth are equivalent to in-person services. In 2016, CMS did not find that the submitted evidence demonstrates a clinical benefit to the patient.
	99358 99359	Prolonged evaluation and management service before or after direct patient care, first hour and each additional 30 minutes, respectively	As indicated in 2015, Medicare does not make a separate payment for these services.
	99444	Online evaluation and management	As indicated in 2008, 2012, 2014, and 2016, this is a noncovered service because it is inherently non-face-to-face and the language of the descriptor indicates that the service could be for noncovered entities, like guardians.
	99490	Chronic care management services	This service can be furnished without the beneficiary's face-to-face presence and using any number of non-face-to-face means of communication.
	99605 99606 99607	Medication therapy management services provided by a pharmacist, initial 15 minutes, new patient; initial 15 minutes, established patient; each additional 15 minutes, respectively	These are noncovered services under the Physician Fee Schedule.[a]
	No code provided	All evaluation and management services, telerehabilitation services; and palliative care, pain management and patient navigation services for cancer patients	The requests did not identify specific codes being requested, and two of the requests did not include evidence of any clinical benefit when the services are furnished via telehealth.

Source: GAO analysis of Federal Register Notices for Medicare Telehealth Services. | GAO-17-365

[a]Medicare pays for physician and other health professional services based on a list of services and their payment rates, called the Physician Fee Schedule.

Appendix IV: Telehealth and Remote Patient Monitoring Reimbursement and Use in Selected State Medicaid Plans

To better understand how telehealth and remote patient monitoring are used in Medicaid plans, we selected a sample of six states—Connecticut, Illinois, Kansas, Mississippi, Montana, and Oregon—to include in our review, and interviewed Medicaid officials from each of those states. We selected states that provide variation in geography, physical size, percentage of rural population, and other factors related to coverage and reimbursement for health care services.

The Centers for Medicare & Medicaid Services does not limit telehealth and remote patient monitoring use in Medicaid, thus reimbursement and use vary by state. The six states had a range of restrictions for the use of telehealth. For example, Illinois requires a medical professional be present with the patient receiving care at the originating site, while Oregon does not require anyone to be with the patient who is receiving care, at what is known as the originating site. More details on the use of telehealth and remote patient monitoring by selected state are included in table 7.

Table 7: Reimbursement and Use of Telehealth and Remote Patient Monitoring in Selected State Medicaid Programs

State characteristics[a]	Reimbursement of telehealth and remote patient monitoring	Use of telehealth and remote patient monitoring
Connecticut Small 12 percent rural Primarily fee-for-service	As described in state documentation, Connecticut passed a law effective July 1, 2016, for coverage under the Medicaid program for telehealth services that are (1) clinically appropriate to be provided by means of telehealth, (2) cost effective for the state, and (3) likely to expand access to medically necessary services for Medicaid recipients for whom accessing appropriate health care services poses an undue hardship. A Connecticut official told us that currently, Connecticut reimburses for provider-to-provider consults via secure electronic messaging, and does not reimburse for any other telehealth or remote patient monitoring services.	A Connecticut official told us that the state has considerable health resources and proximity to specialists, both in Connecticut and in neighboring states, and thus has less need for telehealth use.
Illinois Medium 12 percent rural Primarily managed care	As described in state documentation, Illinois requires telehealth patients to be at an originating site with a physician or licensed health care professional or other clinician present. A physician's office, podiatrist's office, local health department, community mental health center, and outpatient hospitals are allowed as originating sites. Allowable providers of telehealth are hospitals, physicians, advanced practice nurses, podiatrists, federally qualified health centers, rural health clinics, and encounter rate clinics.[b]	Illinois officials told us telehealth is used frequently for psychiatric care.

Appendix IV: Telehealth and Remote Patient Monitoring Reimbursement and Use in Selected State Medicaid Plans

State characteristics[a]	Reimbursement of telehealth and remote patient monitoring	Use of telehealth and remote patient monitoring
Kansas Large 26 percent rural Primarily managed care	As described in state documentation, Kansas does not limit reimbursement based on patient location and allows reimbursement for home-based telehealth. Kansas also does not limit the providers who can offer telehealth services. Kansas officials told us they reimburse for some remote patient monitoring services, such as monitoring of blood pressure, blood glucose, and weight.	Kansas officials told us that telehealth is a valuable tool, especially in supporting emergency room staff in hospitals without a level I or II trauma center nearby.[c] The state has some experience with remote patient monitoring through a pilot project, which ran from September 2007 to June 2010 and, according to a Kansas report, reduced the rate of emergency department utilization.
Mississippi Medium 51 percent rural Primarily managed care	As described in state documentation, Mississippi reimburses for telehealth services that are medically necessary and would otherwise be covered in an in-person setting. Mississippi requires that telehealth be delivered in a live, interactive audiovisual format and does not reimburse for other types of services, such as telephone and email communication. Mississippi reimburses for telehealth services provided in specific originating sites.	Mississippi officials told us they began reimbursing for telehealth and remote patient monitoring in January 2015. Officials told us they focus their use of telehealth on serving high-cost, high-use beneficiaries.
Montana Large 44 percent rural Primarily fee-for-service	According to state officials, Montana does not restrict the use of telehealth. They started reimbursing for originating site fees in 2014, and have increased the number of sites where they provide an originating site reimbursement fee since 2014. Officials told us that they do not reimburse for remote patient monitoring.	Montana officials told us the state does not have any medical schools and has limited access to specialists. As such, telehealth services are important to providing patients with access to specialty care.
Oregon Large 19 percent rural Primarily managed care	As described in state documentation, Oregon reimburses for medically appropriate covered telehealth services within the patient's benefit package. In its definition of "telemedicine," Oregon does not further specify restrictions on originating sites or provider types.	Oregon officials told us they see telehealth and remote patient monitoring as tools to be used by Oregon's coordinated care organizations (CCO) when appropriate for delivering quality, value-based care.[d]

Source: U.S. Census Bureau data, state documents, and interviews with state officials. | GAO-17-365

Note: The term "originating site" refers to the location where the patient is located while receiving a telehealth service.

[a]State size refers to the geographical size of the state and is based on U.S. Census 2010 data. Large states are from the largest third of states by size, medium states are from the middle third, and small states are from the smallest third. Rurality, the percentage of population living in a rural area, is based on U.S. Census 2010 data.

[b]Encounter rate clinics are health care providers actively participating in the Illinois Department of Healthcare and Family Services' Medical Assistance Program as an encounter rate clinic as of July 1, 1988; or, a clinic operated by a county with a population of over three million.

[c]According to the American Trauma Society, trauma center levels (I, II, III, IV, or V) refer to the kinds of resources available in a trauma center and the number of patients admitted yearly. The categorization of trauma center level varies from state to state (including distinctions of adult and pediatric centers). A level I facility is capable of providing total care for every aspect of injury, and a level II trauma center is able to initiate definitive care for all injured patients, while lower levels may not be able to offer as comprehensive of care.

[d]As described in state documentation, Oregon defines a CCO as a network of all types of health care providers (physical health care, addiction and mental health care, and sometimes dental care providers) who have agreed to work together in their local communities to serve people who receive health care coverage under Oregon's Medicaid plan.

Appendix V: Selected Associations' Rating of the Significance of Factors that Affect Telehealth and Remote Patient Monitoring

Through an administered data collection instrument, officials from six associations representing providers and two associations representing patients identified, and rated the significance of, factors that encourage—and barriers that limit—the use of telehealth and remote patient monitoring in Medicare.[1] Officials were asked to respond from the perspective of their association, specifically from a provider or patient perspective, depending on the association.[2]

Figures 4 and 5 show how provider and patient associations rated the significance of factors that encourage the use of telehealth and remote patient monitoring in Medicare. Figures 6 and 7 show how provider and patient associations rated the significance of barriers to the use of telehealth and remote patient monitoring in Medicare.

---

[1] For the purposes of this report, telehealth refers to clinical services that are provided remotely via telecommunications technologies, while remote patient monitoring is a technology to enable monitoring of patients outside of conventional clinical settings, such as in the home.

[2] A representative of the payer association we spoke with told us that it did not have sufficient time to survey its members and could not complete our data collection instrument without doing so. Therefore, we reported separately the payer association's views on factors that encourage the use of or are barriers to telehealth and remote patient monitoring.

123

Appendix V: Selected Associations' Rating of the Significance of Factors that Affect Telehealth and Remote Patient Monitoring

Figure 4: Significance of Factors That Encourage the Use of Telehealth in Medicare, According to Selected Provider and Patient Associations

Factor that encourages telehealth use	Provider associations						Patient associations	
	A	B	C	D	E	F	G	H
Alleviation of provider shortages/scheduling problems	●	●	●	●	◉	●	◐	●
Convenience for the patient	◐	◐	●	●	◉	◐	●	●
Cost reduction	●	◐	⊗	●	◉	◐	●	◐
Coverage of services	⊗	●	●	●	◉	●	◐	●
Emerging Medicare payment structures or waivers	◐	●	◐	◐	◉	⊗	⊗	◉
Enabling the use of emerging technology	◐	○	●	◐	◉	⊗	⊗	⊗
Health Resources and Services Administration telehealth grant programs/other federal initiatives	◐	○	⊗	●	◉	⊗	⊗	⊗
Improving or maintaining quality of care	●	◐	●	●	◉	○	●	●

● A very significant factor that encourages use
◐ A somewhat significant factor that encourages use
○ A factor that encourages use, but not a significant one
⊗ Not a factor that encourages use
◉ Did not respond

Source: GAO analysis of a data collection instrument completed by six associations that represent providers and two associations that represent patients. | GAO-17-365

Appendix V: Selected Associations' Rating of the Significance of Factors that Affect Telehealth and Remote Patient Monitoring

Figure 5: Significance of Factors That Encourage the Use of Remote Patient Monitoring in Medicare, According to Selected Provider and Patient Associations

Factor that encourages remote patient monitoring use	Provider associations						Patient associations	
	A	B	C	D	E	F	G	H
Alleviation of provider shortages/scheduling problems	●	⊗	●	◉	●	⊗	●	●
Convenience for the patient	◐	⊗	●	◉	●	◐	●	●
Cost reduction	●	◐	●	◉	●	⊗	◐	●
Coverage of services	●	●	●	◉	●	⊗	◐	●
Emerging Medicare payment structures or waivers	●	◐	◉	◉	◐	⊗	⊗	◉
Enabling the use of emerging technology	◐	⊗	●	◉	●	⊗	⊗	⊗
Health Resources and Services Administration telehealth grant programs/other federal initiatives	◐	⊗	○	◉	◐	⊗	⊗	⊗
Improving or maintaining quality of care	●	●	●	◉	●	◐	●	●

● A very significant factor that encourages use
◐ A somewhat significant factor that encourages use
○ A factor that encourages use, but not a significant one
⊗ Not a factor that encourages use
◉ Did not respond

Source: GAO analysis of a data collection instrument completed by six associations that represent providers and two associations that represent patients. | GAO-17-365

Note: Remote patient monitoring is a technology to enable monitoring of patients outside of conventional clinical settings, such as in the home.

Appendix V: Selected Associations' Rating of the Significance of Factors that Affect Telehealth and Remote Patient Monitoring

Figure 6: Significance of Barriers to the Use of Telehealth in Medicare, According to Selected Provider and Patient Associations

Barrier to telehealth use	Provider associations						Patient associations	
	A	B	C	D	E	F	G	H
Concern regarding quality of care	⊗	◐	⊗	▨	▨	◐	●	◐
Cost increase or inadequate payment	●	●	⊗	▨	▨	●	⊗	●
Coverage of services	●	●	○	▨	▨	●	▨	●
Cultural factors[a]	◐	⊗	⊗	▨	▨	◐	●	●
Infrastructure requirements[b]	◐	◐	⊗	◐	▨	○	●	●
Pace of changing technology	◐	○	⊗	⊗	▨	⊗	●	⊗
Privacy and security concerns	◐	◐	⊗	●	▨	⊗	⊗	●
Professional licensure issues	◐	◐	●	▨	▨	◐	⊗	◐
Provider/patient training requirements	⊗	◐	⊗	▨	▨	○	●	●

● A very significant barrier
◐ A somewhat significant barrier
○ A barrier, but not a significant one
⊗ Not a barrier
▨ Did not respond

Source: GAO analysis of a data collection instrument completed by six associations that represent providers and two associations that represent patients. | GAO-17-365

[a] Cultural factors may include language and technological literacy, among others.
[b] Infrastructure requirements may include access to broadband internet, imaging technology or peripherals, and wireless communications systems, among others.

Appendix V: Selected Associations' Rating of the Significance of Factors that Affect Telehealth and Remote Patient Monitoring

Figure 7: Significance of Barriers to the Use of Remote Patient Monitoring in Medicare, According to Selected Provider and Patient Associations

Barrier to remote patient monitoring use	Provider associations						Patient associations	
	A	B	C	D	E	F	G	H
Concern regarding quality of care	⊗	●	◎	◎	⊗	⊗	◐	●
Cost increase or inadequate payment	●	●	◎	◎	●	◐	◐	●
Coverage of services	●	●	◎	◎	●	◐	◐	●
Cultural factors[a]	◐	⊗	◎	◎	⊗	⊗	●	●
Infrastructure requirements[b]	●	○	◎	◎	⊗	●	●	●
Pace of changing technology	◐	◐	◎	◎	⊗	⊗	◐	⊗
Privacy and security concerns	◐	○	◎	◎	○	⊗	⊗	●
Professional licensure issues	●	⊗	◎	◎	●	⊗	⊗	◐
Provider/patient training requirements	◐	◐	◎	◎	◐	◎	●	●

● A very significant barrier
◐ A somewhat significant barrier
○ A barrier, but not a significant one
⊗ Not a barrier
◎ Did not respond

Source: GAO analysis of a data collection instrument completed by six associations that represent providers and two associations that represent patients. | GAO-17-365

Note: Remote patient monitoring is a technology to enable monitoring of patients outside of conventional clinical settings, such as in the home.

[a]Cultural factors may include language and technological literacy, among others.

[b]Infrastructure requirements may include access to broadband internet, imaging technology or peripherals, and wireless communications systems, among others.

Appendix VI: Medicare Valuation of Remote Patient Monitoring

Remote patient monitoring refers to a coordinated system that uses one or more home-based or mobile monitoring devices that transmit vital sign data or information on activities of daily living that are subsequently reviewed by a health care professional. This process can enable providers to closely track a patient's condition and provide earlier intervention to potential problems.[1] According to a report by the Agency for Healthcare Research and Quality, remote patient monitoring has been shown to produce positive outcomes, such as reduced hospitalization, when used as a part of care management for chronic conditions such as diabetes and congestive heart failure.

A June 2016 report by the Medicare Payment Advisory Commission (MedPAC) found that Medicare covers some services through its Physician Fee Schedule that involve remote monitoring of a patient.[2] For example, MedPAC's analysis of 2014 Medicare data found that the agency spent $119 million on remote cardiac monitoring services for 265,000 beneficiaries. While remote patient monitoring is used in Medicare, there are concerns about how to establish accurate valuations for some of these services' Medicare payment rates in the Physician Fee Schedule. To identify these concerns, we collected documentation from and interviewed associations representing provider, patient, and payer

---

[1] Monitoring programs can collect a wide range of health data from the point of care, such as weight, blood pressure, blood glucose, blood oxygen levels, and heart rate.

[2] Medicare Payment Advisory Commission, Report to the Congress: Medicare and the Health Care Delivery System, (Washington, D.C.: June 15, 2016). MedPAC noted that Medicare also covers many services under the Physician Fee Schedule that involve a provider's remote interpretation of a diagnostic test. For example, a hospital can perform an imaging study on a patient and transmit the images electronically to a radiologist to interpret the images in another location. Medicare pays for physician and other health professional services based on a list of services and their payment rates, called the Physician Fee Schedule.

Appendix VI: Medicare Valuation of Remote Patient Monitoring

associations.[3] We also reviewed documentation and conducted interviews with Centers for Medicare & Medicaid Services (CMS) officials.

CMS—the agency within the Department of Health and Human Services that administers the Medicare program—values remote patient monitoring services in the same way it values other physician services—by setting payment rates primarily as a result of underlying relative values that CMS assigns to each service.[4] These relative values largely reflect estimates of the level of physician work and the amount of practice expenses needed to provide one service relative to other services.[5] Physician work relative values are based on the estimate of two main inputs: (1) the time the physician needs to perform the service (including pre- and post-service activities, or work performed before and after the service), and (2) the intensity of the service (including the physician's mental effort and judgment, technical skill and physical effort, and psychological stress). Practice expense relative values are based primarily on estimates of (1) direct practice expense inputs, which reflect the clinical labor, medical equipment, and disposable supplies needed to provide a specific service as well as the amount of time for which labor is required and equipment is used, and (2) indirect practice expenses, which generally reflect overhead expenses not associated with a specific service.[6]

---

[3] In conducting our work to describe factors identified as encouraging the use of or creating barriers to remote patient monitoring in Medicare, we collected documentation from and interviewed representatives of associations who represented providers, patients, and payers. To identify these associations, we reviewed relevant documents and literature and conducted interviews to identify general associations, as well as specialty associations that represent common conditions for which telehealth or remote patient monitoring may be used, or could be beneficial, during the course of treatment, such as stroke, congestive heart failure, and mental health. We included 10 associations in our review: 7 associations that represent providers, 2 associations that represent patients, and 1 association representing payers. Not all associations commented on concerns regarding the Medicare valuation of remote patient monitoring.

[4] CMS generates initial relative values for new services and may revise relative values for existing services to maintain their accuracy. The agency generally reviews valuation for several hundred service codes per year, while rates are re-calibrated annually to maintain relativity among the services. CMS reviews the relative values of all physicians' services at least every 5 years.

[5] A third resource, malpractice relative values, accounts for the cost of malpractice insurance premiums of the specialties that perform the service.

[6] For more information about CMS's process for establishing relative values, see GAO, Medicare Physician Payment Rates: Better Data and Greater Transparency Could Improve Accuracy, GAO-15-434 (Washington, D.C.: May 21, 2015).

Appendix VI: Medicare Valuation of Remote Patient Monitoring

Several characteristics of remote patient monitoring services have been identified by some of the selected associations we interviewed as raising challenges to valuation within CMS's methodology, such as the services' personnel and technology, and the operating hours and location of where certain remote patient monitoring services are delivered. Additionally, officials from one provider association noted that some parts of CMS's process for developing Medicare valuation may not consider input from stakeholders most knowledgeable about the technical components of the services.

Personnel. Officials from an association representing certain providers of remote patient monitoring services told us that Independent Diagnostic Testing Facilities frequently perform remote patient monitoring services that include patient diagnostic testing, but some personnel costs may not be recognized in the Medicare valuation methodology because these personnel are not considered clinical staff.[7] For example, personnel involved in remote cardiac monitoring at Independent Diagnostic Testing Facilities include non-clinical administrative staff who the association officials noted are not adequately accounted for in the CMS methodology.

Technology. Officials from this same association also noted that the costs of technology associated with remote patient monitoring may not be fully captured by CMS's valuation methodology. For example, while wearable remote devices only monitor one patient at a time, wireless communication systems—with their hardware and software costs—that can be used to remotely monitor multiple patients at a time are not attributed to an individual patient when considering the direct practice expense inputs.[8] Therefore, this type of equipment is classified within the indirect cost category (with overhead costs), resulting in lower payment

---

[7]An Independent Diagnostic Testing Facility is a diagnostic testing facility that is independent of a physician office or hospital. Its purpose is to furnish diagnostic tests and not to directly use test results to treat a patient.

[8]CMS officials explained that for costs that are not attributable to individual patients, like a centralized monitoring system, the established practice expense methodology considers these costs, like others not attributable to individual services or patients, to be indirect costs. According to officials, they are accounted for through the allocation of indirect practice expense relative value units that would be assigned to the code billed for the monitoring. In contrast, the equipment costs of the monitor worn by an individual patient would be a direct practice expense cost assigned to a particular service code. This direct practice expense cost would serve as an allocator for indirect practice expense relative value units to be assigned to the code (these might represent the costs associated with centralized monitoring equipment).

Appendix VI: Medicare Valuation of Remote Patient Monitoring

rates than if these costs were considered direct costs, according to association officials. Additionally, other unique costs for remote patient monitoring related to technology include such things as the cost of delivering the monitoring device to the patient and the cost of the patient returning the device after the monitoring period has ended.

In addition, technology used to provide remote patient monitoring services can vary among service providers and is evolving, contributing to difficulties in developing valuation for the services. Officials with a payer association said there is variation among the type of devices the patient or provider must possess or that must be installed in the patient's home to carry out remote patient monitoring, such as motion sensors to determine if a patient has fallen or the components that transmit biometric information such as blood pressure or weight back to the monitoring site. Officials with a second provider association noted that remote patient monitoring technology continues to evolve, and for such newly-developed technology there is not a consensus in how to use and charge for the multiplicity of delivery models, including the range of services and procedures.

Hours of operation and location. Some remote patient monitoring may require a monitoring facility to operate 24 hours a day, 7 days per week. An association representing certain providers of remote patient monitoring services noted that Medicare's valuation methodology, which CMS officials stated was designed for and primarily applies to services furnished in standard physician offices during business hours, may not fully incorporate costs associated with maintaining operations outside of standard business hours and in non-physician office settings, such as at Independent Diagnostic Testing Facilities or other types of remote monitoring centers.

Knowledgeable stakeholders. CMS works with a committee established by the American Medical Association (AMA)—the AMA/Specialty Society Relative Value Scale Update Committee (RUC)—three times a year annually to review a subset of physicians' services, identified in part by CMS and in part by the RUC, to develop recommendations to CMS on the resources needed to provide those specific services. RUC members generally represent physician specialty societies, such as those for

Appendix VI: Medicare Valuation of Remote Patient Monitoring

cardiology, family medicine, and internal medicine.[9] However, for services such as the cardiac monitoring services that are widely provided by Independent Diagnostic Testing Facilities, representatives from Independent Diagnostic Testing Facilities do not serve on the RUC and do not officially participate in the RUC process as advisors regarding these services, according to officials with the association representing certain providers of remote patient monitoring services.

CMS response to cited concerns. CMS officials agreed that the payment rates that result from the application of the current Medicare methodology may reflect relative resources for services furnished in the typical physician office rather than other locations. Officials said that they use CMS's annual rulemaking process for setting payment rates for the Physician Fee Schedule to address services, such as remote patient monitoring, that vary from the usual service delivery model.[10] CMS officials said this process affords members of the public an opportunity to recommend codes to be considered for revaluation if they believe the services are inappropriately valued. Some examples CMS officials cited include the following:

- In revisions to the Physician Fee Schedule for calendar year 2016, CMS increased the input price for patient worn telemetry system equipment, which is a factor in establishing the payment rate for cardiovascular telemetry transmitted to a remote attended surveillance center for up to 30 days. In response to a request received in a public comment period during the annual Physician Fee Schedule rulemaking, CMS increased the price from $21,575 to $23,537 to account for the unique properties of the equipment, including its use 24 hours per day and 7 days per week for an individual patient over several weeks and its use primarily outside of a health care setting.

- CMS has developed codes within the Physician Fee Schedule that describe the non-face-to-face care management services that include

---

[9]The RUC members are supported by physician representatives who are responsible for coordinating with their respective specialty societies to develop relative value recommendations to present to the RUC.

[10]Each year CMS publishes proposed and then final rules setting out revisions to payment policies under the Physician Fee Schedule, which include relative values for existing services and for new services as well as opportunities both for public comment on these proposals and for requests from interested parties regarding payment rates for Medicare services.

Appendix VI: Medicare Valuation of Remote Patient Monitoring

interactions furnished through communication technology. These non-face-to-face services are associated with managing the particular needs of patients and are furnished over the course of a calendar month.

Appendix VII: Examples of Telehealth and Remote Patient Monitoring in Medicare Models and Demonstrations

The Patient Protection and Affordable Care Act created the Center for Medicare & Medicaid Innovation (Innovation Center) within the Centers for Medicare & Medicaid Services to test innovative payment and service delivery models to reduce Medicare, Medicaid, and state Children's Health Insurance Program expenditures while preserving or enhancing the quality of care.[1] The Innovation Center also supports Medicare demonstration projects, which study the likely impact of new methods of service delivery, coverage of new types of services, and new payment approaches on beneficiaries, providers, health plans, states, and the Medicare trust funds. The Innovation Center has organized the models and demonstrations into seven categories. Table 8 shows the seven categories and for each provides a description and an example of how a model or demonstration within that category may use telehealth or remote patient monitoring.[2]

Table 8: Centers for Medicare & Medicaid Services' Innovation Center Categories and Examples of Potential Telehealth and Remote Patient Monitoring Use in Models or Demonstrations

Innovation Center category	Category description	Example of a model or demonstration that can use telehealth or remote patient monitoring
Accountable care	Accountable Care Organizations (ACO) and similar care models are designed to incentivize health care providers to become accountable for a patient population and to invest in infrastructure and redesigned care processes that provide for coordinated care, high quality, and efficient service delivery.	Next Generation ACO: This model allows beneficiaries to receive telehealth services at home and in urban areas.
Episode-based payment initiatives	Under these models, health care providers are held accountable for the cost and quality of care that beneficiaries receive during an episode of care, which usually begins with a triggering health care event—such as a hospitalization or chemotherapy administration—and extends for a limited period of time thereafter.	Bundled Payments for Care Improvement models 2 and 3: These models remove geographic limitations on the use of telehealth services.
Primary care transformation	Advanced primary care practices—also called medical homes—utilize a team-based approach, while emphasizing prevention, health information technology, care coordination, and shared decision making among patients and their providers.	Independence At Home Demonstration: This demonstration requires practices to have the ability to use remote patient monitoring and mobile diagnostic technology with their patients.

[1] Pub. L. No. 111-148, §§ 3021, 10306, 124 Stat. 119, 389, 939 (codified at 42 U.S.C. § 1315a).

[2] For the purposes of this report, telehealth is defined as clinical services that are provided remotely via telecommunications technologies, while remote patient monitoring is a technology to enable monitoring of patients outside of conventional clinical settings, such as in the home.

Appendix VII: Examples of Telehealth and Remote Patient Monitoring in Medicare Models and Demonstrations

Initiatives focused on the Medicaid and CHIP populations	Medicaid and the state Children's Health Insurance Program (CHIP) are administered by the states but are jointly funded by the federal government and states. Initiatives in this category are administered by the participating states.	Medicaid Incentives for the Prevention of Chronic Disease: This model included grantees that use telehealth to reach participants dispersed through a large region.
Initiatives focused on the Medicare-Medicaid enrollees	Individuals enrolled in both Medicare and Medicaid (the "dual eligibles") account for a disproportionate share of the programs' expenditures. According to the Center for Medicare & Medicaid Innovation, a fully integrated, person-centered system of care that ensures that all their needs are met could better serve this population in a high quality, cost-effective manner.	The Initiative to Reduce Avoidable Hospitalizations among Nursing Facility Residents: This model includes a participant that plans to use telehealth to provide after-hours telehealth services when needed.
Initiatives to accelerate the development and testing of new payment and service delivery models	Many innovations necessary to improve the health care system are expected to come from local communities and health care leaders from across the country. By partnering with these local and regional stakeholders, the Centers for Medicare & Medicaid Services intends to help accelerate the testing of new models.	The Frontier Community Health Integration Project Demonstration: This demonstration includes testing the use of telehealth in critical access hospitals.
Initiatives to speed the adoption of best practices	The Center for Medicare & Medicaid Innovation is partnering with a broad range of health care providers, federal agencies, professional societies, and other experts and stakeholders to test new models for disseminating evidence-based best practices and significantly increasing the speed of adoption.	The Million Hearts Initiative: This initiative includes information for providers about how they may be able to be paid for at-home blood pressure monitoring devices, and additional information on potential remote patient monitoring use.

Source: GAO analysis of Centers for Medicare & Medicaid Services documentation. | GAO 17-365

Note: Remote patient monitoring is a technology to enable monitoring of patients outside of conventional clinical settings, such as in the home.

Appendix VIII: GAO Contact and Staff Acknowledgments

GAO Contact	Carolyn L. Yocom, (202) 512-7114, yocomc@gao.gov
Staff Acknowledgments	In addition to the contact named above, Karen Doran, Assistant Director; Sarah Resavy, Analyst-in-Charge; Luke Baron; Muriel Brown; Krister Friday; Monica Perez-Nelson; and Helen Sauer made key contributions to this report.

GAO's Mission	The Government Accountability Office, the audit, evaluation, and investigative arm of Congress, exists to support Congress in meeting its constitutional responsibilities and to help improve the performance and accountability of the federal government for the American people. GAO examines the use of public funds; evaluates federal programs and policies; and provides analyses, recommendations, and other assistance to help Congress make informed oversight, policy, and funding decisions. GAO's commitment to good government is reflected in its core values of accountability, integrity, and reliability.
Obtaining Copies of GAO Reports and Testimony	The fastest and easiest way to obtain copies of GAO documents at no cost is through GAO's website (http://www.gao.gov). Each weekday afternoon, GAO posts on its website newly released reports, testimony, and correspondence. To have GAO e-mail you a list of newly posted products, go to http://www.gao.gov and select "E-mail Updates."
Order by Phone	The price of each GAO publication reflects GAO's actual cost of production and distribution and depends on the number of pages in the publication and whether the publication is printed in color or black and white. Pricing and ordering information is posted on GAO's website, http://www.gao.gov/ordering.htm. Place orders by calling (202) 512-6000, toll free (866) 801-7077, or TDD (202) 512-2537. Orders may be paid for using American Express, Discover Card, MasterCard, Visa, check, or money order. Call for additional information.
Connect with GAO	Connect with GAO on Facebook, Flickr, LinkedIn, Twitter, and YouTube. Subscribe to our RSS Feeds or E-mail Updates. Listen to our Podcasts. Visit GAO on the web at www.gao.gov and read The Watchblog.
To Report Fraud, Waste, and Abuse in Federal Programs	Contact: Website: http://www.gao.gov/fraudnet/fraudnet.htm E-mail: fraudnet@gao.gov Automated answering system: (800) 424-5454 or (202) 512-7470
Congressional Relations	Katherine Siggerud, Managing Director, siggerudk@gao.gov, (202) 512-4400, U.S. Government Accountability Office, 441 G Street NW, Room 7125, Washington, DC 20548
Public Affairs	Chuck Young, Managing Director, youngc1@gao.gov, (202) 512-4800 U.S. Government Accountability Office, 441 G Street NW, Room 7149 Washington, DC 20548
Strategic Planning and External Liaison	James-Christian Blockwood, Managing Director, spel@gao.gov, (202) 512-4707 U.S. Government Accountability Office, 441 G Street NW, Room 7814, Washington, DC 20548

Please Print on Recycled Paper.

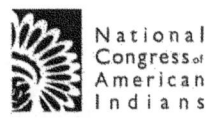 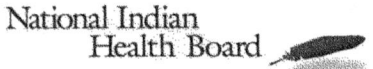

TESTIMONY BEFORE THE HOUSE COMMITTEE ON SMALL BUSINESS; SUBCOMMITTEES ON AGRICULTURE, ENERGY, AND TRADE AND HEALTH AND TECHNOLOGY JOINT HEARING TITLED "21ST CENTURY MEDICINE: HOW TELEHEALTH CAN HELP RURAL COMMUNITIES"

**TESTIMONY OF:
THE NATIONAL CONGRESS OF AMERICAN INDIANS and
THE NATIONAL INDIAN HEALTHE BOARD**

July 27, 2017

On behalf of the National Congress of American Indians and the National Indian Health Board, we submit testimony for the record for the hearing entitled "21st Century Medicine: How Telehealth Can Help Rural Communities" that took place July 20, 2017. We recognize the great potential that telehealth has for rural communities, and as advocates for rural communities, we ask the Committee to consider Indian Country in discussions regarding Telehealth.

As national organizations, the National Indian Health Board (NIHB) and The National Congress of American Indians (NCAI) advocate for Tribal Nations throughout the United States on issuing impacting tribal communities, including broadband deployment and health care issues. We aim to ensure that the trust responsibility is upheld by the Federal Government when Federal Agencies create policies that impact Tribal Nations.

Rural issues are Indian Country's issues, and we see Telehealth as a way forward for Rural Indian Healthcare. Telehealth has great potential to address the health issues that persist in Indian Country. The Federal Governments' trust responsibility to provide healthcare to American Indians and Alaska Natives should most certainly include telehealth efforts. Indian Reservations and Alaska Native Villages are in some of the most rural and remote areas of our country and because of this, American Indian and Alaska Native people should be considered in discussions these rural telehealth issues.

The Indian Health Service (IHS) within the Department of Health and Human Services administers healthcare to Tribal Communities and upholds the Federal Government's Trust Responsibility to Indian Tribes. One of IHS's most glaring problems is the recruitment and retention of qualified professionals. Attracting qualified physicians, nurses, and specialists is extremely difficult in rural America, Indian Country included. We believe that promoting Telehealth within the Indian Health Service, in coordination with the Federal Communications Commission and US Department of Agriculture, will address this glaring issue by allowing quality professionals the flexibility to operate their business while reaching more patients in the Indian Healthcare system. The potential for telehealth in Indian Country should definitely be addressed by Congress.

The Federal Government's Role in Indian Health Care

The Federal Government carries out its trust responsibility to Tribal Nations by providing healthcare to members of Federally Recognized Indian Tribes through the Indian Health Service (IHS) and other federal programs. The Indian Health Service, an agency within the Department of Health and Human Services is a healthcare provider that serves American Indian and Alaska Natives. IHS is a health service delivery system for approximately 2.2 million American Indians and Alaska Natives who belong to 567 federally recognized tribes in 36 states.

Many Federal agencies and offices outside of the Indian Health Service have worked towards the same goal of providing for better health outcomes in Indian Country. Agencies include the U.S. Department of Veterans Affairs (VA), the Substance Abuse and Mental Health Services Administration (SAMHSA), the Administration for Children and Families (ACF), Administration for Community Living (ACL) and U.S. Department of Agriculture Rural Development. Upholding treaty and trust obligations for Indian health is not just a responsibility of IHS, but a trust obligation of all federal agencies that provide health care or implement health related programs.

Lack of Broadband Infrastructure

There are many difficulties in deploying broadband in rural Tribal communities. As the Federal Communications Commission noted in its 2016 Broadband Progress Report, 68% of rural tribal communities lack access to broadband[1]. The FCC has made efforts to address the digital divide that persists in Indian Country, but the lack of broadband deployment in Indian Country continues to affect Indian Health.

In addition, over 1.5 million people living on Tribal Lands lack access to broadband. According to the FCC's 2016 Broadband Progress Report, 41% of Americans living on Tribal Lands and 68% of people living in rural Tribal Lands lack access to high speed internet, compared to the national average of 10%. Some states with the largest telehealth potential have the lowest rates of broadband adoption on Tribal Lands.

The lack of broadband does not only impact healthcare providers' ability to support telehealth and telemedicine; it inhibits a patient's ability to research his/her own health. For 1.5 million people living on Tribal Lands, searching the internet for symptoms, doctors or insurance benefits is simply not an option. While 90% of Americans enjoy the benefits of high speed internet, 68% of Americans living on rural Tribal Lands do not.

Approximately 75% of IHS sites are located in areas defined as 'rural' by the FCC. These rural sites pay a higher percentage of their operating budget than urban locations on monthly circuit costs. When bandwidth upgrades are required, rural IHS sites are frequently asked to fund the capital costs of these upgrades. These projects can take years to complete. In some cases, telecommunication providers are not able to offer any upgrade options for IHS locations.

However, large numbers of IHS facilities do not currently have sufficient bandwidth to offer telehealth and related services. Approximately 50% of the IHS sites are still depending on circuit connections based on one or two TI lines (3 Mbits). Their circuits are constantly saturated with staff experiencing slow response times when using traditional IT applications. The addition of telehealth and mobile health services is not an option at these locations. Services like this are critical in rural communities where recruitment and retention of medical professionals is continually a challenge.

Congress should authorize the Federal Communications Commission to coordinate with the Indian Health Service on addressing Telehealth in Indian Country.

---

[1] 2016 FCC Broadband Progress Report

Lack of Broadband Access on Tribal Lands by State
Data is specific to populations living on Tribal Lands

State	People without Broadband	Percentage of Population	State	People without Broadband	Percentage of Population
Arizona	162,382	95%	Wisconsin	13,042	33%
Alaskan Villages	128,638	49%	Minnesota	12,047	33%
New Mexico	108,604	80%	Colorado	11,875	87%
Montana	40,944	65%	North Carolina	8,910	99%
Oklahoma	36,739	42%	Nevada	7,563	72%
California	29,052	51%	Nebraska	6,393	85%
Idaho	27,666	95%	Oregon	5,517	64%
Utah	24,919	78%	New York	5,472	41%
North Dakota	19,295	80%	Kansas	4,955	100%
South Dakota	19,261	32%	Michigan	4,265	13%
Washington	17,104	13%	Mississippi	2,895	38%
Wyoming	13,202	48%	Florida	1,762	51%
National Average	33.9 million	10%	All Tribal Lands	1.5 million	41%

All above data from the Federal Communications Commission's 2016 Broadband Progress Report-Appendix G

Existing Telehealth Programs in Indian Country

Indian Country has seen a very successful utilization of a variety of telehealth technologies and services, especially regarding behavioral health. However, these successes were achieved on a largely regional basis, driven by visionary leaders in particular communities, with various and not reliably sustainable funding sources. As outlined above, the *IHS has not yet been systematically resourced to establish either a sustainable telehealth infrastructure or governance program* that would prioritize resources in accordance with identified need, establish and promote best practices, and formally evaluate and report on successes and issues.

Telemedicine has allowed Tribal Nations to dramatically improve access to care, accelerate diagnosis and treatment, avoid unnecessary medivacs and expand local treatment options. Program managers have noted that when communities adopt tele health programs, their patients like it and the community wishes to expand telehealth to other programs.

The Indian Health Services' Tele-Behavioral Health Center for Excellence

The IHS Tele-Behavioral Health Center of Excellence (TBHCE) was established in 2008 to provide behavioral health services across the country through real-time (synchronous) video connections.

The IHS Tele-Behavioral Health Center of Excellence (TBHCE) program managers report the following benefits:

1. Patients are **2.5 times more likely** to keep their tele-psychiatry appointments than in-person psychiatry sessions;
2. in FY2013, IHS patients avoided more than 500,000 miles of travel, which translated into over $305,000 in savings for the consumers; and
3. in FY2013, patients saved an estimated 16,450 hours of work or school that would otherwise have been missed to travel for appointments.
4. Native Veterans are more likely to participate in tele behavioral health programs at their local IHS clinic rather than tele health or in person treatment at the closest VA clinic[2]
5. Increased access to specialists and Emergency Services

The TBHCE is operating in 9 IHS Service Areas and at 25 sites. Program managers have reported great successes in the Oklahoma Area for behavioral health and wound care in addition to dermatology and nutrition success in the Phoenix area. However, there are 12 IHS Services Areas and over 300 different sites in the Indian health system – meaning, there are a significant number of Tribal Nations who are unable to access the services provided by the TBHCE. A further expansion of this program, as well as an expansion of broadband and telehealth infrastructure as a whole, is greatly needed to improve access to quality and culturally appropriate behavioral health services for all American Indians and Alaska Natives.

One major impact Telemedicine can have on the Indian Health Service is the benefit of recruiting and retaining professional healthcare staff. The Indian Health Service has historically seen difficulties in recruiting and retaining qualified professionals due to the rural and remote locations of IHS facilities. With Telemedicine, IHS professionals who already understand the health issues of a particular community can stay connected to that community if they move away or relocate. Telemedicine allows for an innovative new way to keep qualified professionals connected to Tribal Communities.

IHS Telehealth Contract in the Great Plains Region

In 2016, the Indian Health Service awarded $6.8 million in telemedicine services to Avera Health to serve American Indian and Alaska Native patients in the IHS Great Plains Area[3]. Because of the vast landscape and remote nature of Tribal communities in the Great Plains Area, emergency services are much more difficult for IHS clinics to address. This contract is providing additional emergency medical services as well as allowing for patients to see specialists in behavioral health; cardiology; maternal and child health; nephrology; pain management; pediatric behavioral health; rheumatology; wound care; ear, nose and throat care; and dermatology.

The outcomes of this program have been positive, however the limited funding has not yet allowed for the Great Plains region to reach its full telehealth potential. Additionally, while this necessary investment to address urgent quality of care issues in this particular Service Area is beneficial, we urge that equal investments be made across Indian Country. Other Service Areas suffer similar issues of poorly resourced facilities and lack of capacity to implement telehealth services.

---

[2] Native Americans have served in the U.S. Armed Forces in greater numbers per capita than any other ethnic group in the United States.
[3] Indian Health Service awards $6.8 million telemedicine services contract to Avera Health, Press Release, https://www.ihs.gov/newsroom/includes/themes/newihstheme/display_objects/documents/IHSPressRelease_Telehealth-Award_09202016.pdf

USDA Rural Utility Service

The Rural Utility Service within the US Department of Agriculture administers telehealth grants through two major programs: the Distance Learning and Telemedicine (DTL) Program and the Community Connect Program. Federally Recognized Tribes are eligible for funding under these grants, and many non-tribal recipients do allocate small portions of funds to neighboring Indian Communities. However, the RUS programs that address telehealth in Indian Country do not sufficiently fund or address the potential for telehealth on Reservations. In January 2016, the Government Accountability Office released a report titled "TELECOMMUNICATIONS: Additional Coordination and Performance Measurement Needed for High-Speed Internet Access Programs on Tribal Lands"[4] which called for better coordination between the FCC and USDA when addressing broadband on Tribal Lands. The FCC is not coordinating well with USDA or HHS on addressing telehealth in Indian Country.

Successful Tele Health Programs in Indian Country

Alaska Federal Health Care Access Network

The Alaska Tribal Health System (ATHS) has relied on telehealth programs to deliver care for more than 20 years. The largest program, the Alaska Federal Health Care Access Network, has been operating since 2001 and has been installed in 250 sites in Alaska. Almost two-thirds of these sites are staffed by Community Health Aides/Practitioners in small Native villages. When first implemented in 2001, internet connectivity was largely unavailable in these village clinics. The Alaska Federal Health Care Access Network created new, innovative technologies that would capture images and patient data for transmission and consultation at other distant sites. Now, the clinical staff, the primary care doctors and specialty doctors can see in real time what is being entered into the patients' medical record. This has greatly improved medication management, reduced hospital re-admittance, increased patient safety and brings a sense of security for all who manage the patients' care. Additionally, in Alaska, the use of telemedicine for audiology and ear, nose and throat (ENT) services not only cut down wait times for Alaska Native patients, it saved consumers and estimated $8-10 million in patient travel costs.[5] The FCC's Universal Services Fund (USF) subsidy program was a large contributor to the expansion and development of telehealth in Alaska Native villages.

Care Beyond Walls and Wires: Telemedicine Home Health Monitoring Program

The Care Beyond Walls and Wires program at Northern Arizona Healthcare, is a telemedicine-based, home-health monitoring program that has significantly improved the health of most participating patients, reduced emergency room visits and hospital admissions and readmissions, and decreased the length of stay for those who still require hospitalization. This program originated in 2011 through a pilot program through the National Institutes of Health Office of Public and Private Partnerships. Northern Arizona Healthcare agreed to conduct a pilot project involving 50 patients that targeted individuals who lived in Supai, a Tribal community located at the bottom of the Grand Canyon. Patients were each given a scale, blood pressure monitors, and pulse oximeters as well as smart phones and solar powered chargers, as many of the participants did not have electricity within their homes. The relationships and sense of security many of the participants developed were reported to have improved health outcomes and reduced unnecessary hospital visits because healthcare professionals could monitor and prevent complications while patients were at their own homes.

---

[4] GAO Report "TELECOMMUNICATIONS Additional Coordination and Performance Measurement Needed for High-Speed Internet Access Programs on Tribal Lands." January 2016.
[5] The Success of Telehealth Care in the Indian Health Service, American Medical Association Journal of Ethics December 2014, Volume 16, Number 12: 986-996. Howard Hays, MD, MSPH, Mark Carroll, MD, Stewart Ferguson, PhD, Christopher Fore, PhD, and Mark Horton, OD, MD

Recommendations

We ask the Congress to consider Indian Country when addressing rural health and moving forward on this issue. To better serve the health needs of Indian Country, and to fulfill the Federal Government's trust responsibility, we recommend the following policies:

Increased Coordination between the Federal Communications Commission, US Department of Agriculture and the Indian Health Service

NCAI and NIHB recommend that the Congress authorize the FCC, USDA and IHS to coordinate efforts and resources to address Telehealth in Indian Country. Existing programs at all three agencies are attempting to address Telehealth on their own without coordination on outreach, outcomes, best practices or data sharing. Coordination between the three agencies would achieve more efficient use of federal funds, better outcomes, better data, and a better approach to solving health disparities in Indian Country.

Tribal Set Aside in FCC Health Funds

NCAI and NIHB recommend that the Congress authorize at least a 5% Tribal set aside for all healthcare related funding that the FCC and USAC distributes. To reach a set aside of at least 5%, we consider the FCC data in the 2016 Broadband Progress Report. There are 1,573,925 people living on Tribal Lands who lack access to broadband out of 33,981,660 people who do not have access nationally. This equates to 4.6%, and rounding up to 5% for the increased costs associated with deployment on the rural and rugged terrain in Indian Country. Congress has authorized set asides like this for many other federal agencies and programs that address the Federal Trust Responsibility to Indian Tribes.

Increase Data Collection regarding Tribal Telehealth

There is very little public information about the potential, impacts or current landscape of Telehealth in Indian Country. GAO's April 2017 Report titled "Healthcare: Telehealth and Remote Patient Monitoring Use in Medicare and Selected Federal Programs" did not address the Indian Health Service, Medicare or Medicaid telehealth programs in Indian Country or any existing programs that impact American Indians or Alaska Natives. We ask the Committee to call on GAO to work with Federal Agencies to provide reports to Tribal governments and the general public in order to better inform decision-making regarding telehealth moving forward.

Conclusion

We thank you for the opportunity to provide our comments and recommendations and look forward to further engagement with the Committee. Please contact Maria Givens, Policy Analyst for NCAI at mgivens@ncai.org or NIHB's Director of Congressional Relations, Caitrin Shuy at cshuy@nihb.org if there are any additional questions or comments on the issues addressed in these comments.

www.ingramcontent.com/pod-product-compliance
Lightning Source LLC
Chambersburg PA
CBHW070247230526
45470CB00002B/507